Around the Globe in 26point2 Miles

Mary Anne Nixon

Mary Anne Nixon

> *"I always loved running...it was something you could do by yourself and under your own power. You could go in any direction, fast or slow as you wanted, fighting the wind if you felt like it, seeking out new sights just on the strength of your feet and the courage of your lungs."*
> *–Jesse Owens*

> *"I haven't been everywhere, but it's on my list."*
> *–Susan Sontag*

Dedication

*For my mom.
Thank you for teaching me
(and hundreds more!)
to read and love books.*
♥

Around the Globe in 26point2 Miles

Diversity among runners around the world is unlimited, yet the 26point2-mile challenge that each marathoner takes on is universal. Preparation for the marathon can vary in endless ways. What does your fellow marathoner from Japan eat for breakfast the day of her race? How does the Latvian participant incorporate unique cross training ideas into her preparations? In what ways do cultural impacts in Uganda contribute to the outstanding results achieved?

Around the Globe in 26point2 Miles is an exploration of training, racing, and recovery ideas from diverse corners of the world. This book is a collection of shared marathon anecdotes, a destination race guidebook, and a toolkit for runners. The international marathon participants featured share a glimpse into their training lifestyles, and no two approaches are the same. Sift through the stories from around the globe, pick and choose ideas that appeal to you and give them a go. By incorporating marathon preparation tactics from different cultures throughout the world, you can find the perfect combination to enhance your marathon experience.

How this Book Works

I asked international marathoners to partake in 26point2 interviews about what goes into their training, race day, and post-race routines. The standard questions just scratch the surface, as there are overlapping strategies that people use regardless of where they are from. The magic happens when each runner focuses on specific aspects of their training and discloses unique culturally based methods.

The Core Questions used in the interviews are the following:

1. What time of day do you run and why?
2. What do you typically eat before or after training sessions?
3. What is your special, secret training tip?
4. Is there any cultural influence, or something going on in your personal life, that impacts your training?
5. Do you add any other exercise to your marathon preparation for cross training?
6. How long is your marathon training cycle?
7. What do you eat for breakfast on the day of your marathon?
8. What did you eat and drink during the race? At what intervals?
9. Deep thoughts: what was your mental preparation and focus throughout training and on race day? Do you use any outside running "distractions" (such as music, podcasts, running apps, etc.) while running?
10. What does your post-race period look like, both for recovery and celebrating? (Note: The celebration after crossing the finish line can serve as motivation that gets you through training and the race!)

Bonus Question: What should you NOT have done in your 26point2? (Not all runners chose to answer this extra question).

The answers to all core questions are featured in each chapter even though information shared by different runners is sometimes similar. This structure allows the book to serve as a reference and makes it easy to flip back and forth through the ideas in a list form to focus on the topics that appeal to you throughout the marathon training cycle.

Introduction

My pre-race ritual might seem slightly crazy. Piping hot and naturally sweet, baked sweet potato fries are almost like eating warm toffee. Eating this comfort food at 6:00 a.m. is not typical, but it became a habit I loved before heading out to races when I took up more competitive running in recent years.

The use of the term "competitive" to describe my running is deserving of the largest quotation marks possible because I only run for the following reasons:

- To explore new places;
- To visit familiar places at different times of the day or as the seasons change throughout the year;
- To commute home from work in an interesting and healthy way;
- To connect with nature or bustling urban energy;
- To feel amazing after finishing a run.

However, a few years ago, I began to participate in road races to shake things up a bit. I figured I could either do my standard river runs along the Guadalquivir in Sevilla, Spain, where I was living or try something new and check out the surrounding villages, each with its distinct feeling. The best way to do this was by visiting when these pueblos were hosting races. On these festive days, the entire small-town population comes out and there is a feeling of excitement in the air. Rows of small kids line up on the race route for high-fives, curious old ladies look down from their balconies, and local bands burst into music to infuse the runners with energy.

Running through these villages is a fantastic way to explore them and offers the bonus of discovering local eats and the opportunity to meet new people while sampling them. Huge organic strawberries were available to savor after the finish line in one village, a bubbly garbanzo stew in another, and an enormous paella rice dish, typically big enough to feed the whole town, was found in others.

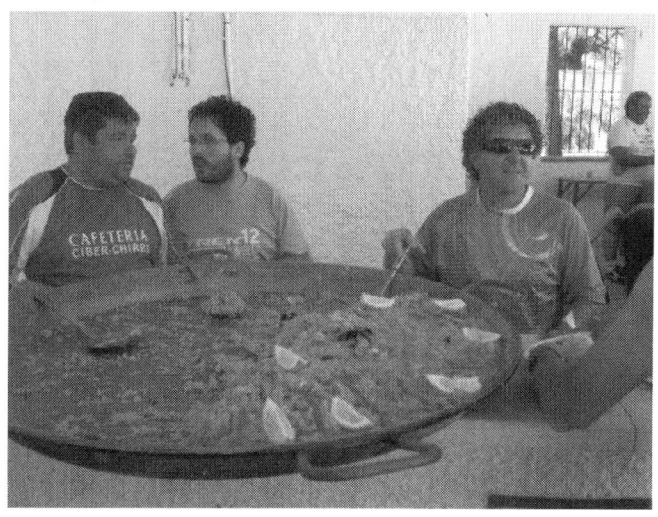

A typical paella served after a race in a small Andalusian village (Photo: M.A. Nixon)

I met new people when I started showing up to the road race scene in southern Spain and connected with a group of amazing runners that overhauled my whole approach to the sport. They were supportive of my new involvement with my old love of running and inspired me in innumerable ways. Over time, this tight-knit community of running buddies evolved into a family on many levels.

It was lovely to connect with these runners on the racing circuit, but it must be noted that whether you show up at any road race in a competitive mindset or not, you are part of an environment that officially takes a close look at numbers. Splits are called out with each passing kilometer, and as you're carried along in a wave of runners, you're subject to a chorus of whiny beeps as GPS watches confirm kilometer crossings. Results immediately flash in large numbers on a screen as you cross the electric finish line mat, and they are always subsequently posted online.

Even if your original motivation was just to do a fun run in an interesting environment and your only dream was to be a gold medal finisher of the line to the beer truck (standard on the Spanish road race circuit because the beer company in question tries to persuade consumers to associate beer with running rather than beer bellies), the final times and rankings are everywhere. They are unavoidable at even the most laid-back race, and numbers are significant. As American rap icon Jay-Z states, "Men lie. Women lie. But numbers, numbers don't lie."

Knowing your running numbers always leads to thinking about how you might improve them. The finishing times reflect progress and accomplishments, so it's reasonable to want to look into the factors involved, including training, diet, and recovery, among a wide array of other components that might increase the odds of hitting that ever-elusive PR (personal record) race time.

In my case, the top pre-race ritual revolved around baked sweet potatoes, no matter how uncommon they might be for breakfast. For me, they are easy to digest and provide a steady wave of energy. With the addition of Spanish olive oil and flaky sea salt, they are delicious.

It turns out I was not the only runner into sweet potatoes. During the summer Olympics, I caught a bit of a television interview with Jamaican runners as they trained on their home island. These phenomenal athletes mentioned a yam/sweet potato variant that was a staple of their training diet. They thought it supported their excellent running performance. Feeling shocked, I whole-heartedly agreed with the Jamaicans and suddenly felt validated by my seemingly random pre-race fueling! This discovery led me to wonder what other amazing runners around the world were eating and exactly what went into their training. How were the cultural preferences that they held impacting their running performance? I felt a strong drive to uncover more of these local customs and try them out for myself in my own running routine.

Not long after this, I was surprised and grateful to be named the poster woman for the Sevilla Marathon. As a result, I was invited to interviews and press events with elite international marathoners that were participating in the race along with me. Meeting these immensely talented runners from far-off countries cemented my curiosity regarding their specific running routines for training, diet, and recovery. I was eager to learn more about exactly what went into their marathon experiences and decided to create *Around the Globe in 26point2 Miles* as a way to explore further.

Read on! Be inspired by the international perspective this book provides, and then lace up your shoes and give some new ideas a try. I wish you happy running!

Why Does This Book Exist?

First and foremost, running is inclusive! It is accessible to people all over, and completing a marathon distance can be a universal goal that runners attempt. People from distinctly different places can use this book to connect based on shared practices. All over the world, we are all more alike than we are different, and this concept absolutely lends itself to running.

There are two groups of people that can benefit from this book: marathon first-timers and veteran marathon runners. Both groups have very different needs, yet these needs also see crossover at times.

Endeavoring to finish the 26point2 for the very first time can provoke a healthy dose of anxiety. There are many unknowns, especially if a person has never taken on a distance quite this long (many popular training plans suggest saving the full length of the marathon for race day). So much time goes into a marathon training cycle, yet there are so many factors that can adversely affect the outcome on race day.

I had mild stress dreams in the weeks leading up to my first marathon. They ranged from taking a wrong turn and veering off the marathon course to being stuck in a long bathroom line (at a churro stand no less since the race I was preparing for was in Spain!) and watching the minutes, and runners, pass by as the dream version of myself waited in slight panic. And this is for a laid-back runner that puts zero pressure on herself! My only marathon goal ever is to do my best while having a great time. Yet stress and nervousness are real no matter how high or low the stakes are, and these emotions can seep into your waking life as well.

Simply gathering information about the unknown diminishes anxiety surrounding an event and can lead to positive feelings while preparing for it. The 26point2 interviews in this book all provide a glimpse into varied marathon experiences. These may (or may not!) overlap with what a new marathoner encounters throughout his or her journey, but just learning how others experience a marathon in advance is a proactive way to find comfort while preparing for a daunting new adventure.

***

> *"Only those who will risk going too far can possibly find out how far they can go."*
>
> *–T.S. Eliot*

***

Highly experienced long-distance runners can also discover new tangible ideas in this book. A marathon training cycle, like anything else, can evolve into something tedious and dull if no effort is made to keep the process fresh. The many training, racing, and recovery ideas found here provide an injection of energy to a tired routine and can help to keep burnout at bay while logging miles. Some ideas may not be appealing at all, while others could become necessary tweaks that even highly seasoned marathoners might add to their plans

Additionally, if a reader is struck by an experience described among these pages, this book could inspire new running adventures in far-off places. Curiosity can spark and eventually become a destination running adventure enabling real-life cultural exchanges.

I chose the marathon distance for this book due to its historical significance and the value it holds as a common thread that connects runners all over the world. While the 26point2 is the focal point, runners of all levels, from 5K joggers to ultra-marathoners, can benefit from the shared knowledge found among these pages.

Notes

It's essential to consult a physician to get training ideas approved before beginning any new exercise endeavor. While the information in this book has been carefully gathered, no responsibility is taken for the correctness found within. This book has both metric and imperial units of measurement since international runners refer to both miles and kilometers (km); all conversions are approximate. *Around the Globe in 26point2 Miles* is a venue for shared experiences and recognizes that all runners, even within the same culture, are unique and can have widely different realities. No experience described here can translate into a blanket statement about any culture. This is simply a space where marathoners contribute what has been true for them.

The 26point2 Interviews

Mile 1. Janelle W. from USA
Mile 2. Queenie M. from Uganda
Mile 3. Mihnea D. from Romania
Mile 4. Julio A. from Ecuador
Mile 5. Diane H. from USA
Mile 6. Baláz S. from Hungary
Mile 7. Sandeep H.A. from India
Mile 8. Johanna W. from Austria
Mile 9. Lia P. from Honduras
Mile 10. Jesper F. from Denmark
Mile 11. Julio M.C. from Spain
Mile 12. Alastair N. from South Africa
Mile 13. Christine D. from USA
Mile 14. Togz T. from the Philippines
Mile 15. Sarah R. from the UK
Mile 16. Ben V.Z. from South Africa
Mile 17. Kristin S. from USA
Mile 18. Ina V. from Romania
Mile 19. Iván F.R. from Spain
Mile 20. Jean-Marie W. from Luxembourg
Mile 21. Željko Š. from Croatia
Mile 22. Diana D. from Latvia
Mile 23. Peter H. from Australia

Mile 24. Becky W. from USA

Mile 25. Emmanuelle G. from France

Mile 26. Mary Anne N. from USA

Mile 0.2 Juan S. from Taiwan

Mile 1: Around the World in Running Shoes
Janelle W. from USA

I was delighted to make the acquaintance of Janelle W. and get a glimpse inside of her expat lifestyle. When you live like Janelle, there is truly never a dull moment. She has made a variety of countries all around the world her home and no matter where she is, she always finds ways to make marathon training a priority. Janelle was born in the United States but is now a running citizen of the world after participating in uncountable international races. She literally could not tell me the number of countries she has run in, in places ranging from Tanzania to Cambodia.

Since Janelle has lived in many of the foreign countries she has raced in, she is able to provide rich background stories about what works for local running, including things like traditional foods that can be incorporated into a marathon training diet, pollution contingency plans, and personal safety strategies. Through her international running, she has also discovered uplifting inspiration and joy from unexpected sources.

Read on to find out what it's like to log running miles around the world and fill your passport with exotic stamps as you go.

1. What time of day do you run and why?

Typically, Janelle aims to get in an early morning workout before the working day begins. What that workout consists of, however, varies depending on where she is living. "In Beijing, I would often have to change my running plans at the last minute if the AQI (Air Quality Index) was too high. My running buddy and I would do stairs instead, or treadmill workouts."

Finding alternatives to outdoor workouts is a necessary reality in places that face air pollution. Making plans to implement effective replacement workouts is key to finding a way around this challenge. When your workout options are limited, it is a good opportunity to add indoor options such as strength training, yoga, or other cross training that runners sometimes go to great lengths to avoid.

2. What do you typically eat before or after training sessions?

Even while living and traveling all over the globe, it is often possible to eat familiar staples. Many foods have become quite widespread and are not challenging to find in out-of-the-way places. "Beans and eggs are usually a go-to since everywhere I've lived has them locally." When living or traveling abroad, finding an indispensable item that works for you and then locating a reliable source that consistently sells it is imperative.

Beyond the basic staples, there are some unique local meals and snacks that Janelle has come to rely on in different parts of the world. She's made training an immersive food experience and at the top of her list are the enthusiastically recommended Beijing dumplings. The ones from Beijing are often pan-fried and boiled. They are delicious, and Janelle feels that the standouts are the potato and leek variety. "They fill you up without feeling heavy, and most are a nice balance of carbs and protein." To add to the deliciousness of this balanced snack, Janelle appreciates the convenience that Beijing dumplings offer, as they are portable and simple to eat on the go.

Janelle's hydration needs, and how she meets them, depend on where in the world she's running. In hotter climates, she adapts and increases her electrolyte intake considerably. "Malaysia and Tanzania — SO MANY ELECTROLYTES! I was constantly rehydrating with coconuts or Nuun tablets."

She goes on to say that "Nuun tablets were recommended by one of my friends who is an Ironman athlete. They ship easily and are affordable. Plus, the flavors aren't too sugary." Since Janelle has traveled the world and tried out a wide range of different options, it's worth taking note of which products she singles out as the best!

Coconut water is also a popular option for rehydration that Janelle uses. It offers runners a clean and light flavor with a potassium-rich boost of electrolytes. Janelle says that coconuts were readily available in many places she's run, including Kuala Lumpur, where, "You could buy them at the store, pop in a straw, and just drink!"

3. What is your special, secret training tip?

Janelle's biggest tip for training in a new country is: "Join a group! I always try to find one as it's a great way to meet people, have a community, and get tips on living in a foreign land." When she moves to a place and no such group has formally existed, Janelle is proactive and initiates a new running club herself. The running buddies often evolve into friends that help her to navigate new cultures.

4. Is there any cultural influence, or something going on in your personal life, that impacts your training?

"Running isn't common in many of the places I've lived, so I'm often very aware of my surroundings. Pregnancy (two times) impacted my training. Where I was living, it was frowned upon for a woman to move around while pregnant, much less work out! I always run with only one earbud in, for safety, and carry my phone in a hidden waist pouch in case I need help." It's essential to develop both a thick skin against critical comments and a heightened sense of awareness when running as a foreigner.

5. Do you add any other exercise to your marathon preparation for cross training?

While Janelle includes swimming and HIIT (High-Intensity Interval Training) exercises in her cross training, she feels that Pilates is the best complement to running as it makes the areas that runners need to work on a focal point. Pilates focuses on core muscles, the IT band, hip flexors, and gluts, and Janelle strongly advocates its injury-reducing benefits. She also noted that adding Pilates to her running during her two pregnancies seemed especially beneficial for her overall wellbeing and post-birth recovery.

6. How long is your marathon training cycle?

As a dedicated distance runner, Janelle generally has a very strong foundation. When a marathon date is on the horizon, she simply begins a gradual increase from her regular workout schedule. Janelle does this mostly through longer weekend runs but realizes that life, including work, family, and travel, can easily get in the way of even the best intentions. She therefore just slowly adds to her normal workouts during the three months leading up to the race the best she can.

7. What do you eat for breakfast on the day of your marathon?

Wherever she is in the world, Janelle sticks to a tried and trusted basic breakfast on race day: bananas and peanut butter. Peanut butter is a powerhouse energy spread that is often misunderstood in countries outside of the US — I have heard it referred to as peanut pâté! However, the combination of protein and fat it offers in a convenient and portable form is ideal for energy before a big event.

8. What did you eat and drink during the race? At what intervals?

As far as the aid stations at marathons around the globe, Janelle has seen it all, including emptied-out tables of food and drinks. Therefore, she has a strategy for hydration that is as simple as it is brilliant. This runner carries a water bottle with her, and if she finds an aid station with drinks available, she'll drink some (about every 30 minutes or so). If there is abundant water for all participants, Janelle will also take the time to fill up her empty bottle and take it with her. "You never know if or when you will have something coming!" she says. Janelle also brings along some type of gummy candy and the previously mentioned Nuun tablets to her races.

9. Deep thoughts: what was your mental preparation and focus throughout training and on race day? Do you use any outside running "distractions" (such as music, podcasts, running apps, etc.) while running?

Although Janelle listens to music or podcasts during training, on race day things unfold differently. She makes it a point to soak up the experience of running in a unique environment. "During a race, I just try to enjoy it first, especially if it's a destination race. I love to stop and take pictures, sometimes to just take a break or to remind myself how lucky I am to be able to do this."

If there aren't any spectators around to cheer her on, Janelle will listen to music for motivation. In some places around the globe, running for fun or fitness is not a common practice. Marathoners have noted that sometimes striding through a village or town, even on a race day, can be met with curious stares rather than cheers. Having music available can provide an upbeat alternative focus.

10. What does your post-race period look like, both for recovery and celebrating? (Note: The celebration after crossing the finish line can serve as motivation that gets you through training and the race!)

This question is where Janelle induces envy due to the fabulous post-race options she has discovered around the world. What she does depends on where she is, but the vibe is always celebratory, and activities range from mimosas and massages to sun and pool time. Janelle will always organize a place to go for special meal afterward as well. But the main thing she looks forward to seeing at the end of her race is her personal crew of cheerleaders. "I love seeing my kids at the finish line and letting them wear my medal."

Bonus Question: What should you NOT have done in your 26point2?

Don't show up empty-handed to your race. It's a smart idea to bring along extra food and drinks. "On the whole, I'm always amazed at how many races that I've done will have NOTHING to eat when you finish. That can be tough, as I'm usually starving, so **I now always try to bring food since there's really never any guarantee**."

There are many standouts among Janelle's international races:

China: You might find a sea of identical T-shirts at a Chinese race. It's a popular concept for all racers to show up in the official event T-shirt. This country, according to Janelle, also gets the prize for most thoughtful hand-outs at aid stations, including wet sponges.

Cape Town, South Africa: "Granted they are in a water crisis, but at the race I did there, they had these neat water pods instead of cups that you bit into. I thought they were novel and smart. Also, there is an AMAZING cheering/running culture there."

Japan: "There are so many other runners there, and it seems like the running culture is well established. There are great big parks, and it's easy to run in the cities."

Tanzania: Delays for the start of race time are the norm, but you will perhaps be entertained while waiting. "Music is big before the race, on the streets made by fans cheering you on and IN the race itself. Expect lots of local music and full-on singing/stomping/group concerts during the race. This is amazing, but it's also impossible to get around the herd of chanting runners." Race organization, or the lack thereof, may be frustrating in Tanzania, but this aspect appears to be improving. "Running seemed to be developing locally with passion as many local groups train and race together — especially groups of women."

Malaysia: Races here often feature very creative and thoughtful routes which take you through beautiful parks, scenic roads, and even jungles! When running in the jungle, Janelle shared that it's best to use trail shoes. "Jungle paths are just as you might think…a little crazy, often mismarked, but exciting. For that reason, I switched over to trail shoes when I lived in Malaysia." Even in some cities, she uses her trail shoes, as so many sidewalks and urban streets feature uneven terrain.

One of Janelle's experiences that resonated with me took place in Cambodia, where she raced at the religious site of Angkor Wat among its dramatic temples. Her words speak for themselves:

Cambodia: "This was one of my favorite places to race. The energy of the people was incredible. During the Angkor Wat race, I just remember landmine victims in old-school wheelchairs racing alongside us with the biggest smiles." The crowd support was incredible. People bestowing generous smiles on the runners lined the streets. Janelle was taken aback by how much everyone delighted in the moment, especially the young fans. "There were so many kids; I think the average family has seven kids, and the entire race is flooded with kids having a blast. It was probably my favorite race and place."

Janelle shared with me that she wished she had written down more about her marathon experiences as she has such an incredible variety of them from all over the globe. I also wish she had, but I'm grateful for the impressions she was able to share here. I have no doubt that Janelle's expat adventures on the run will continue and more memories will follow!

**

Janelle W, from USA, has run in dozens of countries around the world including USA, Cambodia, China,

Japan, Malaysia, South Africa, Tanzania, and the UK

Mile 2: Don't Stop Him Now

Queenie M. from Uganda

It is hard to find a sport more inclusive and accessible than running. Very little equipment is needed (or none at all if you ask the barefoot running contingent!) and you don't need a highly specialized area to train in. **Running can also be a powerful tool to unite people and build communities**, as seen with the success of the efforts of marathoner and race organizer Queenie M. Queenie calls upon his international running expertise to organize and manage running events in Uganda. His initiatives serve as an umbrella for charity endeavors, cultural exchanges, and the promotion of fitness and health for Ugandans of all ages.

By organizing events, Queenie connects people of various backgrounds and communities throughout his home country and indeed the world. I was thrilled to learn about these races and spotlight his endeavors that bridge runners and make this accessible sport (and way of life!) more prominent in Uganda.

Queenie is also instrumental in a social running tradition that originated in Malaysia, where he has run in the past. These fun-loving running events known as Hash Runs are running groups with world-wide participation. They entail more or less focus on the actual running depending on who you're talking with, but Hash Runs are always a good time. These meet-ups highlight the social aspect of running and the importance of relaxing and refreshing with a cold drink after a long run. In Queenie's group, the Kampala branch, participants organize post-run meals and beers ahead of time, and pineapple, melon, and water are readily available during the runs. Queenie says, "Some Hash House Harriers are serious runners, and some are just fun people who love their drinks with a little bit of jogging." Regardless of where you fall on the spectrum, the social aspect provides running-related fun for these "drinkers with a running problem" from all over.

It was also great to learn about Queenie's approach to his own races since he's been able to cherry pick from the different ideas he's seen in practice in various countries. Read on to see exactly what Queenie's 26point2 experiences entail.

1. What time of day do you run and why?

Queenie seeks out crisp morning air for his training. He also perceives the air quality in Kampala to be better at that time of day. He tries to make an extra effort to begin his training before rush hour. "The roads are quieter then. Nowadays, people are always in a hurry to take kids to school, so they drive STUPIDLY fast. This makes my running on school days unpleasant!"

Queenie also mentions something that many can relate to: "As I'm getting older, it is harder to wake early in the morning. But when I do, I have a really nice day after a run." The glow given off after getting in an early morning run leads to positive feelings throughout the day.

2. What do you typically eat before or after training sessions?

Queenie opts for a simple yet effective meal plan. He builds his meals around large quantities of fruits and vegetables with some form of carbohydrates, and will then add either meat or fish to that base. Between meals, he'll snack on nuts and bananas, and drink freshly-squeezed juice in addition to plenty of water.

3. What is your special, secret training tip?

While on very long runs, Queenie uses an uncommon rehydration technique that he borrows directly from very small children. "**Oral rehydration salts make for the best sports drink ever, and they are cheap**. This mix is formulated for babies that have sick stomachs, so it is a perfect balance of sugar and salt." This strategy makes sense for a gentle hydration alternative that will be easy on the digestive system.

4. Is there any cultural influence, or something going on in your personal life, that impacts your training?

Queenie has run in many countries. He feels that, "There is plenty to learn or see in terms of culture, depending on where you race. Many things differ from race to race and country to country." He has taken note of the differences to add a few of them to his races where applicable. Since he puts in an enormous amount of time and energy into the organizational side of the marathons he manages, it's no surprise that when he participates, he does the same.

5. Do you add any other exercise to your marathon preparation for cross training?

While not outside of the realm of running, one standout cross training strategy that Queenie incorporates is to add a lot of speed to his marathon training plan. For him, the addition of sprint workouts pays off. This is despite the fact that Queenie is an avid long-distance runner. He even took on the iconic Two Oceans Race, which is a 56 km (35 mile) ultra-marathon that takes place in South Africa and has been named time and time again the world's most beautiful racecourse. The route hugs the peninsula of Cape Town, and the views are stunning.

Even when considering the amount of endurance necessary for such an extensive distance, Queenie is not one to shy away from speed workouts. "I do love a speed session," he declares. He'll do this in the form of interval series, either 10x400 meters or 20x200 meters with one-minute rest periods between the sprints. He believes "**A mixture of speed sessions will help you run well from 10 km to long distance.**"

He also employs a pyramid approach to his speed workouts. The method involves starting with a broad base of distance at a target speed and then working your way up the pyramid by decreasing the distance but increasing the speed. If Queenie wants a really hard training session, he'll do the whole process in reverse and work his way down the pyramid as well, which is nothing short of impressive.

In addition, Queenie has also recently become a fan of spinning and will opt for 90-minute classes to get in an effective yet lower-impact workout that pushes his heart rate. On active rest days, he'll also sprinkle in small doses of yoga and swimming.

6. How long is your marathon training cycle?

Queenie gives himself a period of 12 weeks before a marathon for training. He feels this is enough time for him to work on both his endurance and speed.

7. What do you eat for breakfast on the day of your marathon?

"I am not an early morning eater which has always been a big problem for me before a race, but I eat lots of fruit as that treats my stomach very well!!" He adds that he will sometimes include some bread and pasta as well.

8. What did you eat and drink during the race? At what intervals?

Queenie will drink water throughout the race and add it to the rehydration salts he mentioned before. If he needs a big boost of energy mid-race, he'll have a Lucozade as well. Lucozade is talked about in more detail in Chapter 16 and is popular on the African marathon circuit.

Here Queenie also shares a strategy that was new to me! "I always ask friends to have a 200ml cold beer waiting for me at kilometer 38 [roughly the 23.5-mile mark] — this has always worked for me." That small taste must make for great motivation to get to the glory of the finish line and the post-race celebration to come!

9. Deep thoughts: what was your mental preparation and focus throughout training and on race day? Do you use any outside running "distractions" (such as music, podcasts, running apps, etc.) while running?

"I have been running since childhood, and I've never used any running distractions such as music, etc. As a runner, I always have to focus on my body, breathing, pace, and technique. With music playing, you're never going to feel all these important aspects of your running."

10. What does your post-race period look like, both for recovery and celebrating? (Note: The celebration after crossing the finish line can serve as motivation that gets you through training and the race!)

Perhaps that small taste at kilometer 38 sets the stage of what is to come after Queenie crosses the finish line, which is, according to him, "BEER!" Many runners choose beer over wine or cocktails for a celebratory toast because the body appears to handle it a bit better after a long run. This is due to the higher fluid content it has when compared to the volume of alcohol. Taking a cue from his Hash Runs, Queenie happily anticipates a toast with beer, followed by a good meal with abundant water, to salute his efforts upon completing a 26point2.

After his celebratory meal, Queenie will head off for an ice bath. Even in warmer temperatures, Queenie does not look forward to this part of the recovery, which he claims is excruciating. He does, however, recognize its undeniable benefits.

Queenie's efforts through his organization Activate Uganda have connected Ugandans of many different walks of life with visiting athletes that want to race in a unique and inspiring environment, while also doing something positive for the local communities in which they run. To find out more about Queenie's running initiatives at the premier sports event management organization of Uganda, look to Activate Uganda at www.activateuganda.com.

Beyond races in awe-inspiring settings (at the source of the Nile River, for example), Queenie manages athletics events involving his other interests: trail running, mountain biking, and ultimate Frisbee, where he hopes to usher Uganda into the world championship tournament. "With all my international experience, it wouldn't be fair if I didn't share that with Uganda!" Queenie's energy is contagious, and he is just getting started. Runners that live in Uganda, or are passing through, can join him.

***

Queenie M., from Uganda, has run in Uganda, Germany, Kenya, Japan, Malaysia, the Netherlands, Rwanda, Tanzania, South Africa, and USA

Mile 3: Revitalized Running
Mihnea D. from Romania

If there is an exotic race out there, Romanian marathoner Mihnea D. has probably either done it or is shortlisting it for a future adventure. Mihn has taken on races in iconic places such as the Great Wall of China, and the ancient city of Bagan, in Myanmar, where he did a temple run marathon. He has also done longer races, including a nice little jaunt of about 80km (roughly 50 miles) which started at the Palace of Versailles and ended a few stories up the Eiffel Tower for the *Eco Trail de Paris*.

Mihn has an enthusiasm about running that is contagious, and he likes to add as many adventurous elements as possible to his destination runs. They say that fortune favors the brave, and when Mihn travels to remote places, he is graced with many incredible running experiences. He has also picked up a few tips along the way that he is willing to share, including the recipe for an isotonic running beverage popular in his homeland.

When out on long trail runs while training or racing, Mihn prepares a drink that offers the benefits of an isotonic beverage and all of its ingredients can be found at a farmers' market.

A sports drink (also called an energy drink) is considered isotonic if it has a mix of electrolytes and carbohydrates that is taken up by the body at about the same rate as water. These drinks are ideal for distance runners as they serve two purposes: to quench thirst and provide energy. Mihn's drink, which he has coined "Marathoner's Isotonic," was created to refresh and hydrate while providing an alternative to beverages with artificial ingredients. Isotonic drinks that are often handed out at the refreshment stations at races are made with added colors and artificial flavors, and their neon hues are not typically found in nature! Mihn prefers the natural and simple ingredients seen here:

Marathoner's Isotonic

Ingredients:

Three lemons

Two grapefruits

Two leaves of fresh mint

Water

Ice

Honey (to taste)

Instructions:

Wash and cut up the fruit and put all ingredients into a CamelBak-style hydration backpack. Start to run for at least 20 minutes. As the run progresses, the ingredients will naturally muddle, and the flavors will shine through. Drink as desired throughout the activity. Water and ice can be added as the run continues. Although the original flavors will eventually become somewhat diluted, it will still be delicious and refreshing.

Mihn is highly enthusiastic about his recipe: "Imagine climbing a steep mountain and after 35 km you feel quite thirsty… with no refreshment point or water nearby… then taking a sip of this special drink… you will feel incredibly refreshed and energized. The remaining trek should be no problem. When at a refreshment point, you fill the backpack with more water and the drink continuously mixes itself while running, releasing more flavor!" When it's Mihn and his drink vs. the mountain, all bets are on Mihn.

Mihn has suffered from digestive problems while racing. He believes that his homemade beverage is gentler on his system than highly processed sports drinks.

1. What time of day do you run and why?

"I am not an early bird," Mihn states, and he therefore does not subscribe to the daybreak workouts that so many marathoners choose. He prefers to run in the evenings after work.

2. What do you typically eat before or after training sessions?

Mihn has simple advice here: "During training I eat normally, trying to balance carbs with proteins and fat and proper hydration. If on Sunday there is a race or long training, I try to reduce the consumption of meat and fats the day before and to skip any alcoholic drinks."

3. What is your special, secret training tip?

Mihn noticed that adding an extra stretching session (he now does one before the run and one after running) has a notable impact on his wellbeing.

4. Is there any cultural influence, or something going on in your personal life, that impacts your training?

Mihn faces time constraints due to his work schedule, but he still adapts his running to what suits him. He is very self-aware and knows he won't feel motivated for a long run if he forces himself to get up early and squeeze it in before his job. Mihn simply carves out time later in the day to make running work with his schedule.

5. Do you add any other exercise to your marathon preparation for cross training?

"I get better results if I go swimming regularly and do core strengthening during my training. When I do this, my body is more resistant throughout the marathon effort." He takes care not to overdo it, though. "These extra training sessions must be seen as a secondary goal because doing too many of them can do more harm than good."

6. How long is your marathon training cycle?

Mihn is another year-round marathoner and has no great need to adhere to a strict training cycle. A marathon (often in a far-flung destination) always seems to be right around the corner for him. He sometimes views his 26point2 not so much as a race, but as prep for future mountain trail running adventures.

7. What do you eat for breakfast on the day of your marathon?

Mihn avoids eating before a race or long run because of stomach issues.

8. What did you eat and drink during the race? At what intervals?

Mihn knows the importance of staying hydrated throughout a race and will drink from each aid station. He will grab a banana if they are available and often relies on his unfailing Marathoner's Isotonic.

9. Deep thoughts: what was your mental preparation and focus throughout training and on race day? Do you use any outside running "distractions" (such as music, podcasts, running apps, etc.) while running?

"I do not run with any music or apps, only with my sports GPS watch. I check the watch constantly to monitor my time and pace. Usually, I am focused on my goal, and I just try to clear my mind from stress or bad emotions."

10. What does your post-race period look like, both for recovery and celebrating? (Note: The celebration after crossing the finish line can serve as motivation that gets you through training and the race!)

Wherever he goes, Mihn is the life of the party, and that carries over to post-race celebrations. When he finishes any race, he enthusiastically looks forward to the party to follow.

Rounding out his list of ideal celebratory components are big meals, chocolate, and watermelon! "Also, a big motivation is the finisher medal to add to my collection."

Mihn has an eclectic mix of medals from around the world. Many marathoners greatly anticipate the joy of getting new bling for their collections. I met one racer that even runs full marathons while carrying all the medals she has earned from previous races in the series (76 up to this point!) in a small backpack. Towards the end of the race, she takes them all out to proudly cross the finish line wearing her accumulation of hefty hardware.

Bonus Question: What should you NOT have done in your 26point2?

The main takeaway that Mihn shares here focuses on the days leading up to the marathon, including the night before. "It's never a good idea to have a few beers the day before the marathon, or to eat heavy meals that include a lot of meat...But for some reason, I don't always learn from my mistakes, ha ha!"

I laughed when I read Mihn's response because I have witnessed him making the most of a great party until the sun comes up. If that party happens to be close to a race day, he probably relies even more on his hydrating Marathoner's Isotonic to see him successfully through to the finish line.

***

Mihnea D., from Romania, has run in
Romania, Austria, China, France,
Germany, Italy, Myanmar,
and Spain

Mile 4: Run now, dance later
Julio A. from Ecuador

Julio A. is the social backbone and ambassador of good times of his running club. This is not to suggest that he doesn't take running seriously — he is a tremendously dedicated athlete; so dedicated that he recently branched out from his running achievements to complete a full Ironman triathlon (bravo, Julio!). Making social connections while running is just something he thrives on and for him is as much a priority as reaching his athletic objectives.

This social butterfly attitude extends to Julio's day-to-day life as well. I once asked him how he made the citrus-based *ceviche* and *empanadas* (savory pastries that are beloved in many regions of South America) he served at one of the many dinner parties he hosts. He casually said that he struck up a conversation and made friends with an older woman while waiting in line at the grocery store (as one does!). It turns out that she was a native of Ecuador, where Julio is also from, and she agreed to come over and help him out with his cooking efforts. The results were delicious.

That is a typical day for Julio, and his openness carries over to his running activities. He is based out of a major European city where many international professionals move in and out of town for work. Julio never hesitates to invite a newcomer to train in the Sunday running group where he is a regular. The post-run brunch will find Julio chatting up a storm and guaranteeing everyone has a good time.

Julio's upbringing in Quito, Ecuador, is partly responsible for his extroverted ways. In Ecuador, there is an ethos of spirited social connections and large gatherings of family and tightly knit groups of friends are the norm. Julio now lives abroad, but his philosophy towards interacting undoubtedly has its roots in South America. He notes that back home people typically see their extended family every weekend without fail and connect with their friends at least twice a week. This constant positive engagement with others is key to the friendly vibe that Julio radiates.

Additionally, he says that dancing is mandatory at social gatherings in his home country. I have run into Julio at many parties and even a formal ball. The ball took place in a breathtakingly beautiful palace, but the mood in some of the great rooms was on the stuffy side. Julio definitely took part in livening up the dance floor.

So how does all this relate to Julio's driven attitude towards running and his ability to obtain excellent results? How does the life of the party and curator of memorable moments even manage to find the time to put on his running shoes and train?

Julio normally opts to run as early as possible to clear up the day for any social adventures that might come along. While this choice seems quite obvious in retrospect, it makes great sense in a social context. When put into practice, it eliminates the temptation to skip a workout because a spontaneous social plan pops up. There is no undue deviation from a training plan since miles have already been logged for the day.

1. What time of day do you run and why?

"During marathon training, I prefer to run early in the morning (6:30 a.m.)." Knowing Julio, he might even make a new friend during his early morning run, so the best bet is to leave his schedule free later in the day in case plans come up.

2. What do you typically eat before or after training sessions?

Julio is very laid back about this aspect and does not

overthink the fueling of his training and racing.

3. What is your special, secret training tip?

Julio doesn't complicate things and says his main tip is to **be dedicated and just show up**. He believes in doing something training-related at least once a day.

4. Is there any cultural influence, or something going on in your personal life, that impacts your training?

Julio recalls that about 15 years ago in Ecuador, the concept of running started becoming more popular. At the time, he was beginning his professional career and looked for a hobby in which he could be active after sitting at a desk for long hours, and so he chose running. Because the sport was rapidly gaining popularity, it was good timing for finding new races and training mates (in Julio's case, future friends!).

5. Do you add any other exercise to your marathon preparation for cross training?

Julio believes he derives his strength from years of team sports such as volleyball and basketball and maintains that that base helps him cope with the stress that running marathons places on the body. These days, he combines marathon training with biking and swimming.

6. How long is your marathon training cycle?

Other than lightly increasing the distance of his running sessions, Julio doesn't really employ any special training plan within a set timeframe.

7. What do you eat for breakfast on the day of your marathon?

While this point is of utmost importance to some, Julio doesn't pay too much attention to the fueling aspect of running. At most he simply adds an extra slice of bread to his breakfast on the morning of the race.

8. What did you eat and drink during the race? At what

intervals?

Julio feels that success at an event boils down to hydration. He makes a point to stop at every station on the racecourse to drink. If he's hungry, without giving it too much thought, he'll grab a banana or energy gel or whatever else is offered during the race to get him to the finish line.

9. Deep thoughts: what was your mental preparation and focus throughout training and on race day? Do you use any outside running "distractions" (such as music, podcasts, running apps, etc.) while running?

Julio's easy attitude is most apparent here. "My philosophy is just to have fun. **No one is paying me for participating in a race, so my goal is to get to the finish line feeling happy.**" True to character, he chooses to be present and enjoy the company around him.

***

> *"The reason we race isn't so much to beat each other but to be with each other."*
>
> *–Christopher McDougall*

***

10. What does your post-race period look like, both for recovery and celebrating? (Note: The celebration after crossing the finish line can serve as motivation that gets you through training and the race!)

It should come as no surprise that Julio follows up his race day achievements with friends, celebratory drinks, and good food. I am quite sure that Julio would also attempt dancing despite any potential issues with sore muscles. He never concerns himself with any special recovery techniques or diet modifications after a race. "If you train properly, you should not feel like you need to do anything special afterward."

Not everyone is an extrovert like Julio, but running with a group, joining a club, or finding a running buddy to prepare for a 26point2 makes the journey much more rewarding. There is an indescribable collective energy that comes from being around other runners, and it moves everyone forward effortlessly. Julio knows this and generously looks to share that energy so other runners can benefit and have a great time while doing so.

***

Julio A., from Ecuador, has run in Ecuador, Austria, Croatia, and Spain

Mile 5: How to Reboot
Diane H. from USA

Diane H. is a running machine. During years of athletic endeavors, this American runner and triathlete has evolved to become an elite Ironman contender that earned a slot to compete in the world championships in Kona, Hawaii, USA. When she focuses specifically on the marathon component of her competition, the high level of her athleticism and her dedication to fitness are evident. Diane is willing to invest in new ideas if it means that they will help her come out on top. She borrows practices from running professionals and adapts them to her own particular needs to achieve outstanding results.

Running workouts cause stress on the body, and this holds especially true for long-distance training sessions. Proper recovery is key to reducing injury and overtraining fatigue, and over the years Diane has learned what works best after pushing herself to the limit. One of the tactics that she has found especially effective involves the use of comically large inflatable boots to help her rejuvenate after grueling workouts. These boots cover most of the leg and are used while lying down. They promote circulation and blood flow after a workout, to ultimately reduce soreness, and work by running compressed air throughout the boot chamber. The airflow delivers a massage-like pressure from the sole of the foot to the top of the leg. This concentrated air compression helps to promote the release of lactic acid in the muscles. Many find that after using the boots, recovery time is reduced, and a feeling of calm ensues.

For Diane, it took time to embrace this practice, but once she firmly decided to incorporate the recovery boots into her routine, she discovered that she can't imagine going without them. "I had looked at the boots for years and then the opportunity was right to get them. For two years I've used them after long training days and sometimes multiple times in those days. Otherwise, I use them two times a week because I don't have time for much more." Thirty minutes is the recommended time for an inflatable boot recovery session, so they do require a considerable commitment if used consistently in a routine. (See www.normatecrecovery.com for more information about NormaTec brand boots).

Diane relies on the recovery boots mostly during her peak building phase and before she tapers off from the hard work put into the training cycle. She compares the effects of using them to that of an ice bath. Her typical ice bath system involves, "running a tub of cold water and adding a small bucket of ice. I'll dip in for 20 seconds and then out and repeat." The repeated jumping in and out of the freezing bath doesn't seem quite as appealing as lounging on the couch wearing puffy cartoon boots, so it's a no-brainer which practice Diane chooses to do more often.

Below, Diane spills the tea on how she applies her marathon training to other aspects of her life, such as weight management, connecting with her family, and a vent for her competitive drive.

1. What time of day do you run and why?

As a working mom with kids that also have busy schedules, Diane does her runs in the early morning as often as possible.

2. What do you typically eat before or after training sessions?

There's nothing exotic about Diane's training diet. She turns to basic, well-balanced meals and eats plenty of bananas for snacks.

3. What is your special, secret training tip?

"Lose weight." It's important to recognize that running long distances while over your target weight puts extra stress on joints. Diane turns to the scale to gauge where she should be to feel her best while running. She always aims for a specific weight before a big event so that she can train more efficiently and stave off injury.

4. Is there any cultural influence, or something going on in your personal life, that impacts your training?

Running helps Diane deal with stress and feeds her competitive character. It is encouraging to hear about an athlete, especially a woman, that fosters the need to be competitive at times. Diane should be applauded for bringing this concept out front and center, as this very normal feeling often gets suppressed. A healthy dose of competitiveness does not equate a catty rivalry, and Diane is able to recognize and even embrace this. She turns competition into a game, and in this game she prefers being the hunted, as opposed to being the hunter. "At a race, I'll try to chase people in front of me, but I find it best if I know a contender is behind me. I run better if I'm being chased." Evading her hunter is often what it takes to push the needle of her internal speedometer and achieve an exceptional result.

Diane noticed that she felt this competitive drive while racing among the greats in the elite Kona event, but at the same time, she was able to bask in the glow of simply being present among such phenomenal runners. For Diane, Kona embodied, "So many great aspects, namely being able to compete with such high-caliber athletes from all around the world. There were people out running all hours of the day/night, and communication was done through hand gestures. Being on a course with the pros is awesome." This experience pushes Diane to always strive for more.

Diane also found that sharing her passion with her family has helped her training and provided some memorable moments. Her son joins her runs at times and at nine years old, he was even able to stay on course with her during a long and hilly training run. She admits that on that occasion she rewarded his efforts in the form of a new Lego toy, but it was quite an achievement for him to stick with her! Regarding mixing her kids in with her training, Diane said that at first she'd feel guilty about "dragging them along," but now they are older and more independent, and they claim that they miss joining her on runs. It is clear that she's exposed her children to a healthy and active lifestyle and it's highly likely that she's planted some seeds of interest for them to pursue their own athletic adventures in the future.

***

"This type of lifestyle shouldn't be sacrificed if you have kids, and kids should realize that it's fun and normal and good to make these types of choices."

–Cynthia Arnold (record-setting marathon mom who pushed a triple stroller weighing 185 pounds (84 kilos) while running a 3:11 marathon) as quoted to Runner's World magazine

***

5. Do you add any other exercise to your marathon preparation for cross training?

During her marathon training, Diane turns to swimming and biking to incorporate different muscle groups.

6. How long is your marathon training cycle?

With such a solid base, Diane will train with as little as two months to go before race day and finds that to be enough.

7. What do you eat for breakfast on the day of your marathon?

The protein and carbohydrate power found in the combination of oatmeal with peanut butter is what Diane loves to eat on race day.

8. What did you eat and drink during the race? At what

intervals?

Throughout her 26point2, Diane will ingest gels, water, and drinks with electrolytes (if the weather is hot). She prefers gels that offer a mix of caffeine and amino acids, and she singles out the GU Roctane line, designed for high-intensity, long-duration activities, as her favorite (www.guenergy.com). These vegan gels are notably higher in price than other gels on the market, but they are said to be some of the best available. Additionally, many reviews state that GU Roctane flavors such as pomegranate blueberry or vanilla orange are refreshing without being cloying.

9. Deep thoughts: what was your mental preparation and focus throughout training and on race day? Do you use any outside running "distractions" (such as music, podcasts, running apps, etc.) while running?

Diane likes to track her data as she runs and claims that doing so makes her run faster. She also tries to run on different courses to prevent boredom and keep things interesting. Diane is always looking for new scenery to run through and ideally seeks out wooded areas with rolling hills. In fact, the weekend I met her, she had just discovered a new running trail along river bluffs near a campsite where we were all staying. The impending chill of fall camping, featuring snowflakes in October, did not deter her from extensively exploring a new hilly area that morning.

10. What does your post-race period look like, both for recovery and celebrating? (Note: The celebration after crossing the finish line can serve as motivation that gets you through training and the race!)

Regarding recovery, Diane abides by the saying, "The first 24 hours are the only 24 hours." She looks to get on a massage table as soon after a marathon as possible, even at the venue of the race if massage services are available. Her next priority is "getting lots of rest," and the first thing she'll do the day after a race is a gentle workout consisting of a jog and a light swim.

Bonus Question: What should you NOT have done in your 26point2?

Overtraining is Diane's biggest issue, and after years of fierce competition she has learned to dial the training down when needed. Less means more in the big picture.

After returning home from each major athletic endeavor, you can be sure to find Diane putting in some well-deserved restorative time on the couch in the company of her recovery boots. Being highly competitive doesn't mean underestimating the value of downtime and relaxing moments with family.

***

Diane H., from USA, has run all over USA and Canada

Mile 6: The Change in Terrain Game

Baláz S. from Hungary

I met Hungarian Baláz S. mid-marathon, and we chatted and logged miles through the rolling Slovenian countryside. He was a focused and studied runner, acutely aware of his pace and intent on hitting his time splits. Even so, he was kind enough to talk with me and share how living in Budapest had influenced his marathon training. After I tracked him down post-race, we discussed in more detail how a change in terrain, namely the use of what some believe to be the world's longest rubberized running track, can have a significant impact on marathon training.

Baláz took up running to control his weight. He had tried numerous other things to shed pounds, including cycling to work, swimming, and a highly detailed diet provided by a nutritionist. The needle on the scale, however, refused to budge. For Baláz, running was the most effective way to see results. Once he took up the sport, he immediately began to shape up.

Budapest is home to a long strip of land in the middle of the Danube River called Margaret Island. *Margitsziget*, as the island is known locally, was once a haven for hunters, but it now hosts a small zoo, waterslides, a spa, a Japanese garden, and pop-up events ranging from concerts to cocktail nights. You can access the island by boat, or if you're out for a run, you can go over the ornate Margaret Bridge.

The island is a true urban escape and a way to get in a nature run without ever having to leave the city. The views of Budapest along the river are superb and change dramatically according to time of day or season. Baláz trains there regularly for practical reasons because it is close to home and he appreciates that you can run for miles at a time without any interference from traffic.

One singular feature of Margaret Island is the rubberized race track that hugs the shore of the Danube. It seems to go on forever, but the We Love Budapest website has it measured at 5.3 km (3.29 miles). Some say it is the longest rubberized running track in the world! But even if it's not, it is an impressive, original, and beautiful run to do while immersed in nature in the heart of a European capital city. It is a location that attracts runners at all times of day, all year round.

When Baláz was over his target weight, he started on the track because he felt the surface to be gentler on his knees. As he lost weight, he continued to train on the track (or on a traditional 400-meter track) for different reasons including the practicalities it presented when doing timed series interval workouts. He did mention, however, that when it rains, he finds the track surface on the island to be slippery and so he avoids it.

If you ever make it to Budapest and want to go for a run, Margaret Island is a unique place and should not be missed. Baláz appreciates that the air is fresher there than in the city. When I was there, I relished in the people watching and spectacular views of the Danube with its ships floating by. What made my run truly special, though, was that unique track surface that Baláz mentioned. It puts a noticeable bounce in your stride and makes for a fun run. Alternatively, you could head to a traditional running track and explore how the surface feels different. If you want to experiment with a variety of surfaces to add different dimensions to your runs, try trail runs, beach runs (best in my experience when the sand is packed and flatter near the shoreline at low tide, unless you want to run in loose sand for an added challenge), and runs in the snow.

Budapest is also home to world-famous thermal baths and spas featuring pools of different temperatures for soaking.

So traditional are these pools that it's common to see groups of locals that look like they have been visiting the baths for decades playing chess while relaxing in the therapeutic water. The baths are actually part of the Hungarian health care system and as such, massages, laps in pools, and soaks in the medicinal waters are often prescribed by doctors. I found that they made for an ideal post-run soak in a unique atmosphere, but Baláz thinks that the thermal baths are too crowded. When he goes for a swim, he prefers the low-key swimming pool near his work in the suburbs.

1. What time of day do you run and why?

"It depends on the season. From the middle of autumn until the middle of spring, I usually do my training in the afternoon after working hours. During the hot summer, I prefer to avoid the heat, so I do 70 to 80 percent of my training before work. The only constant exception is my regular interval training, which happens every week on Tuesday afternoon. These are the hardest workouts, and therefore I do these with a running group." **Make setting a weekly date for a tedious training aspect a habit. It's much harder to avoid that workout when it's penned into your calendar**.

2. What do you typically eat before or after training sessions?

"In the mornings I don't eat before training, but after I usually drink some milk, and I have my breakfast at work. During afternoons I make sure not to eat for at least three hours before training. After running in the evening, I usually have dinner, which I try to keep small (some fruit, some cheese, walnuts, and puffed wheat)."

3. What is your special, secret training tip?

Baláz believes it's better to go for distance rather than speed, with the one exception of his weekly interval workout day. He also shares his approach to tapering the week before the race, which he feels works best if you make sure to do shorter runs of about 5 km (3.1 miles) at your slowest possible pace. This strategy should bridge the hard training and the race day while keeping you light and loose.

4. Is there any cultural influence, or something going on in your personal life, that impacts your training?

Baláz's quest for improved health through running was based on data that he came across. "I read an article about the health effects of being overweight, and there was comparative data about how a certain amount of extra weight equates to time of life lost. I do not remember the numbers, but I calculated that my extra weight was equivalent to five to eight years of lost life, so I decided to make a drastic change." Baláz then took up his marathon training.

In an entertaining side note, Baláz also had some motivation from home to participate in his first marathon, just not necessarily in the way one might assume wifely support would look like: "I ran my first half marathon race in April 2017 and my second in August. At the end of August, I asked my wife, "What do you think, am I able to accomplish the Budapest Marathon in the middle of October?" She said, "Definitely not." So basically, she gave me the ultimate motivation, which was to prove her wrong. During that time, I was running around 40 km per week, so I decided to increase it to 50 km, with longer runs on weekends. The result was a marathon finish time of 3:55:53." Motivation can clearly come in a variety of packages!

5. Do you add any other exercise to your marathon preparation for cross training?

In the past, Baláz incorporated strength training into his routine but currently he swims to break up the running. He has participated in long-distance swims, including a long 5.2-km (3.2-mile) challenge across Hungary's beautiful Lake Balaton (which is the largest freshwater lake in Central Europe and is surrounded by picturesque vineyards). He decided after the challenge that he needed less swimming during his marathon training cycle as it was taking too much time away from running.

I understand this concern because every time that I pack up my bag to go across town to the pool and swim, I have to remember a variety of swim accessories, a change of clothes, a towel, flip flops, and shower items. During this process, I always feel a moment of appreciation for how easy it is to simply step out my front door and start a workout when I go for a run. The fact that running involves little more preparation than throwing on a pair of shoes (a step which some runners even skip!) makes it even more rewarding.

6. How long is your marathon training cycle?

Interestingly, Baláz answered this question in terms of distance rather than time. In his response, he broke down his monthly progressive distance plan, which looks like this: month one: 50 km/week (31 miles); month two: 60–70 km/week (37–44 miles); month three: 70–80 km/week (44–50 miles); month four: 80 km/week (50 miles); last two weeks: 40 km/week (25 miles). According to the plan, he dedicates about 4.5 months to his marathon training cycle.

7. What do you eat for breakfast on the day of your marathon?

"Basically I eat the same every time, and it's not a typical runner's breakfast. I eat scrambled eggs with a lot of cheese about three to four hours before the race. Immediately before the race, I usually eat a banana or a muesli bar. I ate this before my first race, and I do not change things that work well."

8. What did you eat and drink during the race? At what intervals?

"I don't drink isotonic drinks. I do not really like the taste. I always drink water during a race, and I have as much as possible. I keep in mind my first rule of thumb, which is: **A**

runner has to drink before they get thirsty. I also usually take a banana, if available, but I don't do any serious planning about what to eat."

9. Deep thoughts: what was your mental preparation and focus throughout training and on race day? Do you use any outside running "distractions" (such as music, podcasts, running apps, etc.) while running?

"I only ran once with music in training, and I did not enjoy it, because my earplug continuously slipped out of my ear. So, I skipped this idea. I did not do any mental preparation. I just try to raise the bar every time and accomplish my goals. I always set an unreachable target for myself." Sheer joy ensues when the "unreachable" target is actually met.

10. What does your post-race period look like, both for recovery and celebrating? (Note: The celebration after crossing the finish line can serve as motivation that gets you through training and the race!)

Baláz gravitates towards sweets to reward his marathon efforts. "After a race I immediately drink and eat things that contain a lot of sugar." Coca-Cola and chocolate top his list of preferred treats.

Bonus Question: What should you NOT have done in your 26point2?

"The biggest mistake to avoid before training or racing is eating too much. This can cause serious and unpleasant situations."

***

**Baláz S., from Hungary, has
run in Hungary, Italy,
and Slovenia**

Mile 7: Jaggery to Boost and Yoga to Ground

Sandeep H.A. from India

I felt fortunate to come into contact with Sandeep H.A., who shares how he benefits by incorporating traditional practices from his homeland India into his running. He originally got into distance running while participating in other sports such as long-distance cycling, trekking, and his preferred "sport" of jumping up and down and screaming while cheering for hours on end at cricket matches; he swears it's a great cardio workout! He eventually became interested in adventure trail running, which later evolved into participation in road races.

According to Sandeep, road races have only become more widely seen over the last 10–15 years in India, and mainly in major urban areas such as Bangalore, Chennai, and Delhi. He was happy to be present in the country as running grew in popularity, and he now lives in Germany and continues to run in road races. Sandeep has varied experience running abroad, but no matter where in the world he runs, he counts on traditional tactics and philosophies from home.

One of Sandeep's go-to energy boosters while running is called *jaggery*. *Jaggery*, also referred to as *gur*, is an unrefined sugar product that is found in India. In a hospitable gesture, it is often served in people's homes in rural villages when guests visit. According to Sandeep, "*Jaggery* is from sugarcane, and I guess it is less processed than other kinds of sweeteners. It tastes both sweet and salty. Since it is in a more natural form, it contains a lot of nutrients including iron." He noted that *jaggery* was traditionally offered to guests that traveled from great distances to remote Indian villages as it reduces fatigue after long trips. Sandeep reasoned that it could be useful for long distance runners as well. "You just need a small piece, like the size of a piece of hard candy. You might not feel anything instantly energetic or special immediately, but soon your fatigue lifts."

Sandeep involves the philosophies of another traditional custom into his running as well, in the connection that he finds with India's 5,000-year-old practice of yoga. Yoga is emblematic of India and most associate the practice with a series of poses that stretch muscles. Sandeep values the physical aspects of yoga, but beyond the postures, he feels that the focus on breath work and mindfulness highlighted in yoga are helpful in the context of running. "I prefer to have minimum support from gadgets during training. You need to listen to your body for injury-free race preparation," says Sandeep. This advice could be taken straight from a yoga instructor. Although Sandeep initially relied on the use of electronic devices and detailed progress charts to adjust his pace and overall training, he eventually learned to listen better to his body, and modify different aspects based on how he felt rather than what the data told him. "I took this advice from yoga. Our bodies have such sophisticated sensors that no other monitoring devices are needed."

He goes on to say that, "Over time I've come to realize that our bodies give us accurate information and adjust themselves accordingly. For example, if you ask ten people to run, each person will have a different posture that suits that individual's physiology. This is a natural tendency. Why would someone run with a posture that feels wrong?" Sandeep is quick to clarify that he considers himself merely a "hobby runner" and that his observation is not professionally informed. Even so, the intuitive element that he uses to improve his running is of value, and so is the perspective he provides in the following questions.

1. What time of day do you run and why?

"In Mumbai, India, of course it's early in the morning, such as 5:30 a.m. or 6:00 a.m. The weather is pleasant only until 7:00 a.m. and then the high humidity in Mumbai makes it very difficult to train. In Mumbai, you cannot run midday. One must get up early to run."

The early morning training option in steamy climates is overwhelmingly popular. Sandeep also used to commute to work on his bicycle to work to add in some cross training. It was a 25-kilometer trip (15.5 miles), and he noted that doing this in his city was only possible because he went against the heavy flow of the often-crazy weekday traffic and therefore felt safer.

2. What do you typically eat before or after training sessions?

Sandeep does not stray too far from his regular diet when training. "I try to keep regular meals with balanced nutrition. I prefer a banana or two before running. For recovery, I like homemade electrolyte drinks consisting of a mix of salt, sugar, and water or *jaggery* with water."

3. What is your special, secret training tip?

Sandeep's tip circles back to his use of the philosophies seen in a yoga practice and the application of them to running. He highlighted the importance of paying attention to your breath as it's an excellent indicator of your exertion level.

4. Is there any cultural influence, or something going on in your personal life, that impacts your training?

"Yes, regarding life circumstances. I feel that the busier the day is, the more motivation I find for training. However, if I have a relaxed day, then I find it hard to motivate myself to train." I was thrilled to read about Sandeep's view because to me, it seemed like a major juxtaposition and as such, it gave me a fresh point to consider. It always seems to me that a hectic day at work slowly leads to a mental tally of reasons (ahem, *excuses*) that can push the needle towards not getting out for a run that day. This is along the lines of, "I'm getting so tired, I need to finish one last bit of work, it will get too dark to run by the time I get out, or it will coincide with dinner plans, etc."

Sandeep, however, counterintuitively reframed this mental argument and decided that **the busier he is, the more he needs and deserves the run after work**. This shift in the paradigm helped me see training from a new vantage point. I internalized the concept and now view a run as a reward for dealing with a long, stressful day, as opposed to one more thing to tick off the list of things to do after work. Bravo to Sandeep for converting a potentially negative situation into a productive mindset.

5. Do you add any other exercise to your marathon preparation for cross training?

"Stretching is a must, and I use cycling, swimming, and hiking for cross training." This is in addition to the athletic level that is apparently needed to be a passionate cricket fan!

6. How long is your marathon training cycle?

Sandeep has an active lifestyle and maintains a high fitness level. In this connection, he employs a relatively short training cycle of about two months leading up to race day.

7. What do you eat for breakfast on the day of your marathon?

"Bananas. Easy to eat. No preparation needed." This is a spot-on summary. The humble and affordable banana is in fact a nutritional powerhouse that many runners turn to. They are sometimes described as nature's PowerBars, and they could not be simpler to eat — ask any toddler.

There is one point to consider, though, when planning on eating this energy-enhancing staple before a 26point2. I have heard of racers running at destination races popping out of their hotels the night before the event to find bananas at their preferred level of ripeness. Although bananas are often available at hotel breakfasts, many complain that they are still green and not as appetizing to eat as a speckled and soft banana. It's better to track down a perfectly ripe banana the day before, and in many places, it's usually not at all hard to find them. In a lot of countries, bananas are even found at convenience stores.

8. What did you eat and drink during the race? At what intervals?

Sandeep extends his practicality to race fueling and opts for energy bars, because as he says, "They are easy to carry." He will also eat bananas and drink isotonic beverages, when available, at the refreshment stations.

9. Deep thoughts: what was your mental preparation and focus throughout training and on race day? Do you use any outside running "distractions" (such as music, podcasts, running apps, etc.) while running?

Sandeep aims to feel present and mindful of his surroundings on race day. He thrives off the energy that live bands and music blasted on the racecourse contribute. "I prefer not to listen to any music during the race day because I like to run with very little on me. I feel free and relaxed, and the music playing along the route helps give me all the adrenaline rush I need."

10. What does your post-race period look like, both for recovery and celebrating? (Note: The celebration after crossing the finish line can serve as motivation that gets you through training and the race!)

Sandeep rewards himself with a Coca-Cola after the race and then immediately goes off to rest. His extended years of running have reduced the level of post-race excitement. "Celebration was certainly there for the first couple of races, but now I have a different routine: Wake up, run, go back home." Immediate rest is certainly well-deserved after completing a race, so there is no shame in skipping the finishing party. Here, yet again, Sandeep listens to his body and responds accordingly to what it needs.

The addition of traditional practices found in India to a forward-thinking racing strategy is valuable. Different techniques can both pick us up and keep us grounded and focused. By incorporating an assortment of ideas, Sandeep has created a formula that works for him wherever he runs in the world.

***

Sandeep H.A., from India, has run in India, Austria, and Germany

Mile 8: Espresso for Express Workouts

Johanna W. from Austria

Johanna W. ran the Vienna City marathon in her homeland of Austria for her 26point2 debut, and her training involved one interesting addition in the form of a steaming beverage in a tiny mug. Espresso is a must for this distance runner, and especially so when consumed in conjunction with her early morning workouts. She aims to do these runs immediately after waking up and before eating breakfast. This practice, called *Nüchternlauf* in German, should be done intermittently. Johanna first heard about the strategy when a sports doctor that works in medical tents at marathons suggested she give it a try.

The closest translation I've been able to find for *Nüchternlauf* is "sober running," and this is clearly a very loose definition. The idea is to get the run in before anything else, so you are "sober" and not weighed down. A cup of espresso, taken with a glass of water before heading out, is however allowed and even encouraged. According to www.datasport.com, "In the morning, after getting up, your glycogen stores are not quite full, and your insulin level is low. According to the theory, if you train in this state, your metabolism will not run in "carbohydrate mode." Instead, the body will use more fat as fuel to train its metabolism. In endurance sports, the more economically the metabolism of fat works, the more carefully the carbohydrate reserves can be used. In order to be able to perform as well as possible for long distances and/or competitions, it makes sense to train the fat-burning metabolism." Opinions on this vary, but the practice works well for Johanna, and she makes it a part of her routine to partake in a quick coffee before heading out.

Coffee is a notably important part of life among my Austrian friends, so this little extra to Johanna's training plan did not get so much as a raised eyebrow from me. It seems that for many Austrians, weekend socializing involves (or revolves around) coffee and cakes. Are you going on a day-long bike ride? Great, but where is the stop planned for coffee and cakes? Visitors coming from out of town? Where's the best café to take them for coffee and cakes? Holiday celebration with loved ones? Sounds wonderful, but who is organizing the afternoon coffee and cakes? I'm guessing that Johanna would enjoy an additional coffee after her *Nüchternlauf* if cakes were also involved.

I am very happy to include Johanna's representation of her homeland, which is my current country of residence, among these pages. Austria boasts postcard-perfect scenery to run in, with highlights including mineral-rich Alpine lakes that take on almost a Caribbean sea color; hills that are truly alive due to their blooming wildflowers at certain times of the year, and a carpet of wild garlic at other times of the year; and the impressive Danube River that is studded with bluffs and apricot trees. Austria's capital Vienna allows runners to use convenient public transport to get to hills made up of stunning vineyards and leafy woods that hug the outer-lying districts. This area actually forms part of the foothills leading to the Alps and grants sweeping views of the city below. Vienna is comprised of about 50 percent green space and boasts a network of unique federal gardens that make for ideal running spots.

Johanna often finds that the beauty of Vienna provides motivation for her to get out for a run. For more information on her marathon training strategies, read on.

1. What time of day do you run and why?

Johanna allows for some flexibility within her running schedule and tends to keep it varied. "During the week, I go for after-work runs, on the weekend I'm all over the map."

2. What do you typically eat before or after training ses-

sions?

While in marathon mode, Johanna will often add extra carbs for lunch and occasionally for dinner as well. She eats figs and dates for energy if she runs midmorning or later in the day. She accompanies all meals and snacks with large amounts of water.

3. What is your special, secret training tip?

This is where Johanna's previously mentioned "*Nüchternlauf* runs" come into play. "I go for short runs of 5 km or less right after getting up, and of course, I drink a small espresso before heading out."

4. Is there any cultural influence, or something going on in your personal life, that impacts your training?

"Yes, my work situation did impact my training. Sometimes I was too tired to go running, so in those instances, I had to force myself to go out." Johanna made this possible, and even enjoyable, by finding the most beautiful running spots for inspiration on those challenging days. Since Vienna is home to numerous palace gardens that are free and open to the public, she often chose manicured landscapes featuring an abundance of striking flowers, sculptures, and fountains. Her resistance to the run always diminished once she was immersed in the stunning scenery. Johanna, and all residents of Vienna, are privileged to have easy access to these grand landscapes.

***

> *"Vienna has baroque gardens you can visit for free…It is not common in Europe; in Germany, England and Italy, you pay to visit the gardens. I see the Bundesgarten [federal gardens] as a living museum."*
>
> *–Austrian Federal Gardens Director Gerd Koch as told to Metropole magazine*

***

5. Do you add any other exercise to your marathon preparation for cross training?

Johanna rounds out her training with occasional sessions of Pilates and light biking. Her Pilates practice positively impacts her running since it enhances balance, stability, and core strength.

6. How long is your marathon training cycle?

Johanna believes that an extensive period of preparation can be incredibly beneficial to the results. "Had I started regular training about six months beforehand, I think I could have done better in the race. For my next marathon in April, I will start my training cycle in October, and follow a much stricter schedule."

7. What do you eat for breakfast on the day of your marathon?

"I ate toast with peanut butter and bananas, tea without sugar, a hard-boiled egg, and had water with a dissolved magnesium tablet (to help avoid muscle cramps during the race)." Before starting the race, she also took some mineral water and white bread with her to the starting area, for light last minute fueling before the pistol fired.

8. What did you eat and drink during the race? At what intervals?

Johanna shared that in addition to water, Coca-Cola, and isotonic drinks, she dissolves gels in water and drinks them. This particular strategy was new to me but sounds interesting to try, especially if you're looking for a specific flavor or ingredient (many gels have caffeine) that is only available in gel form. Johanna aimed to rehydrate at every aid station, and she also ate a banana during the second part of the race.

9. Deep thoughts: what was your mental preparation and focus throughout training and on race day? Do you use any outside running "distractions" (such as music, podcasts, running

apps, etc.) while running?

Johanna doesn't use music or anything else that could distract her from her running performance. Her sole mental tactic was to simply visualize the finish line and anticipate the joy she would feel upon crossing it.

10. What does your post-race period look like, both for recovery and celebrating? (Note: The celebration after crossing the finish line can serve as motivation that gets you through training and the race!)

"I should have done a lot of post-race stretching immediately after crossing the finish line, but I was late to meet with colleagues from work, so I did a tiny bit of stretching and then walked to the nearest *U-Bahn* [subway station]. On Monday morning, I had the worst muscle pain I can remember, and it lasted until Wednesday morning or so. I think that the *Muskelkater* [aching] was a combination of just having completed a marathon enhanced by not having stretched enough after the race."

Johanna also rummaged through her finishers' bag after her 26point2 and sampled its contents, which consisted of a bottle with cold vegetable broth, sparkling apple juice, a protein drink, and some chocolate. It was a somewhat unusual combination of products, but she appreciated all of them.

Bonus Question: What should you NOT have done in your 26point2?

Johanna stopped mid-race for a massage, but in retrospect she would've skipped it because she thinks it had little effect on how her legs felt afterward.

For future marathons, she says she will practice a motion which might seem simple but, as any runner can verify, can be tricky to carry out: picking up and drinking from the cups at the aid stations while in motion. "I can vouch that this is a challenging task." One simple strategy is to fold the lip of the cup to control how fast your beverage pours out.

When Johanna feels a little less motivated to train, she gets encouraged by her beautiful surroundings and of course the extra boost from her *Nüchternlauf*. These things will surely see her through to future marathons.

***

Johanna W., from Austria, has run in Austria, Germany, Italy, Latvia, Luxembourg, the Netherlands, Norway, and Switzerland

Mile 9: Fire on Ice
Lia P. from Honduras

Lia P. is a running enthusiast from Honduras, Central America. Honduras is a country that will always hold a special place in my heart for its captivating natural beauty, simple yet crave-worthy food, and ubiquitous yellow school buses reminiscent of my daily transportation as a kid (although, admittedly, my childhood buses weren't blasting salsa music and didn't have any passengers carrying bags of live chickens). Most of all, Honduras is dear to me because of its warm and welcoming people known as *los Catrachos*. *Catrachos* know how to make the most of life and rise above the many challenges found in this corner of the world.

I was fortunate enough to experience living in Honduras for over two years as a US Peace Corps volunteer, and while I did run at the time, my experiences were completely different from Lia's recent marathon preparation. It should be noted that I was there almost two decades ago and running for fun did not seem to be a widely understood concept, especially in my small mountain town.

Lia's energy and spark for running and life shone through as she answered my questions. Her enthusiasm is contagious and made me feel a pang of desire to get up before 5:00 a.m. to run in the cool air of a Honduran morning among the chorus of roosters before the hot sun breaks. The thought of a traditional *Catracho* breakfast afterward adds even more appeal!

Marathon preparation involves an array of challenges that range from time management to injury prevention to choosing fueling options. Most runners face these issues when preparing for the 26point2. Lia did as well, but she also had extra challenges to consider. During her marathon training cycle, national protests and strikes sometimes made the streets of her area of Honduras unsafe. The demonstrations became increasingly violent, and Lia and her family were affected. There was one intense month that felt especially unsafe to Lia, as widespread unrest blanketed the entire country.

Lia didn't feel comfortable running outside during that time, and her training was reduced to running within the limited confines of her *colonia*, which roughly translates to immediate neighborhood. She felt protected in her familiar surroundings since the neighbors always kept an eye out for her, but she had to make do with a much shorter running route of about 2–3 km (roughly 1.5 miles). She never let this limitation deter her and always kept her fiery drive.

Lia is also the first runner in my interviews that enthusiastically advocates what she refers to as "cryotherapy." Cryotherapy is simply the application of ice to treat tissue lesions. Lia uses ice in the recovery phase of her training after a hard run. Her variation is to submerge her legs in cold water and ice cubes for periods between 3 minutes up to 15 minutes. She is adamant that this is a useful addition to her routine and eagerly encouraged me to try it as well. It's possible that this therapy seems more appealing to those living in tropical climates, so despite Lia's excited insistence, I think I will wait until after a run in a sweltering place to try it out.

While the ice bath technique is nothing new to distance runners, the difference is that many talk about it with unveiled displeasure. It is not usually the first thing on the recovery menu that a runner chooses to order. Yet Lia's sheer energy and cheer regarding everything related to doing what she loves carries over, even to this practice. She radiates a sincere love for all aspects of marathon training. That fire can't be diminished even when submerged in an ice bath.

1. What time of day do you run and why?

"I begin running at around 4:30 a.m. since I need to be at work early. At first, it's hard getting up at that time, but you get used to it when you're doing something you love!" Honduras is generally a very early-rising country. Since the hours of daylight don't vary much throughout the year near the equator (daylight hours are roughly from 5–6:00 a.m. to 5–6:00 p.m. in this region) many Hondurans are up quite early to take full advantage of the daylight. Additionally, the temperatures and humidity can be sweltering in many parts of the country, so the early bird approach can improve productivity. On the weekend, Lia allows herself a bit of a sleep-in and starts her day at 5:00 a.m.

2. What do you typically eat before or after training sessions?

Before a running workout, she usually consumes a bit of apple or orange juice and a small banana. Any size, shape, and class of banana you can imagine are found in abundance in Honduras, which is also known as the Banana Republic. This is quite useful for runners looking for a boost of potassium.

Lia will have a cold drink waiting for her when she returns from her run, and then she will partake in a famous *Catracho* breakfast. I would be remiss not to mention how this meal provides comfort and sustenance on so many levels. When you sit down to a steaming plate of handmade tortillas, fried plantains, beans, eggs and creamy avocado that contrasts crumbly *cuajada* cheese, all with a fresh mug of local Honduran coffee, you will be fully satisfied. "This breakfast will help you restore your energy very quickly," enthuses Lia.

There is an alternative breakfast option that Lia also recommends for people that don't have the time to sit down to a full meal. In this case, a more portable snack called a *baleada* can be a great selection. *Baleadas* can have a lot of similar ingredients as the abovementioned *Catracho* breakfast, but they are served in a large, folded tortilla and can be eaten on the go.

3. What is your special, secret training tip?

While Lia didn't offer a specific tip here, it's clear that her attitude is the foundation of her successful training. Success, to a great extent, hinges upon the attitude you chose to accompany you on any journey.

4. Is there any cultural influence, or something going on in your personal life, that impacts your training?

The strikes in Honduras affected Lia's marathon training plan, but she made the necessary adaptations in order to maintain her training cycle.

She also took many of her drinks in plastic bags instead of cups or bottles. All around Honduras, you can see beverages ranging from water to cola to fresh juices, and yes, even isotonic drinks, served in bags. People can be seen in every town sipping the contents of their bagged beverages through a straw or a small hole bitten off the corner of the bag. Lia found these bags to be quite practical and comfortable for hydration throughout her training and during the 26point2.

5. Do you add any other exercise to your marathon preparation for cross training?

Honduras has changed a lot since I was a resident. Fitness has become increasingly popular and, as a result, gyms and fitness centers have popped up and are in high demand. Lia reports that Cross-fit fitness studios, which feature group training with varied functional movements taken from weightlifting, gymnastics, calisthenics, rowing and more, are now commonly found. Lia reports that incorporating Cross-fit into her marathon training notably strengthened her legs, arms, and core. She shares that her legs felt much more resilient after participating in Cross-fit, and she believes that this helped her avoid injury.

6. How long is your marathon training cycle?

After completing a half marathon in her hometown, Lia felt motivated to take on the full 26point2. She found a marathon that was five months away and used that window of time to train.

7. What do you eat for breakfast on the day of your marathon?

Lia's light breakfast on the big day consisted of a granola bar, half a banana, and a small amount of juice.

8. What did you eat and drink during the race? At what intervals?

Lia did not try anything that was offered at the rest stations because she wanted to stick with what she knew to avoid any possible ill effects. She only had water and Gatorade at 5-km (3 mile) intervals until the last 10 km (6 miles) of her race. At that point, the sun became so oppressive that she feared dehydration. Since she had come prepared with a hydration running belt, she started drinking at each subsequent kilometer.

9. Deep thoughts: what was your mental preparation and focus throughout training and on race day? Do you use any outside running "distractions" (such as music, podcasts, running apps, etc.) while running?

In the weeks leading up to her marathon, Lia made it a point to get in touch with her running friends and listen to as much motivational advice from them as possible. She chose not to listen to music during her race, but she used the Strava app on her phone to track her performance.

10. What does your post-race period look like, both for recovery and celebrating? (Note: The celebration after crossing the finish line can serve as motivation that gets you through training and the race!)

After her marathon, Lia's family and friends that had cheered her on gathered with other runners to have a celebratory lunch near one of Honduras' beautiful golden beaches. When she got home, she made sure to submerge her legs in an ice bath for a full 15 minutes and then took it easy for the rest of the day. The following day was a Monday, so she went to work as normal, but got a massage to relieve her muscle tension after her workday

Bonus Question: What should you NOT have done in your 26point2?

Lia wishes she would've tried to eat some solid food during her training runs instead of just drinking liquids along the way. That way, she would've felt more comfortable eating during her marathon.

Lia's spark for running is so bright that the most accurate way to describe it could be the description of something wonderful exclusively used in Honduras: *cheque-leque*! This distinction only applies to standout things and can absolutely be extended to our exemplary Honduran marathoner, Lia.

***

Lia P., from Honduras, has run in Honduras, Guatemala, and Miami, USA

Mile 10: Becoming a Master

Jesper F. from Denmark

After traveling the globe for ever more interesting places to train and race, Olympic marathoner Jesper returned to his native Denmark to continue breaking records in his career as an elite runner while expanding his focus to include becoming a father and an educator. His multifaceted life is a lot to juggle, and it often pulls him in many directions. Jesper relies on various training strategies he's picked up along the way in order to keep his running in gear.

While chatting with Jesper, he shared a viewpoint that stuck with me: "You become what you do." For example, he may alternate between focusing on very long distances, or sprint splits during his workouts. Alternatively, he might make strength training a focal point. Whatever he pays particular attention to, he ends up becoming (i.e., a more adept distance runner, a runner with a fast kick at the end of a race, or a stronger, more resilient competitor). Determine what to focus your energy on and use this mindset to become that.

"I am in a situation where I have limited time and energy to do everything that is required to perform at my best level. I see it as a scale that can be tipped in one direction or another, for instance: mileage vs. intensity. I normally choose to run over other training options, because it is the most specific component of training, and **you become what you do**."

Namely, Jesper wants to become a Master. Soon he will be competing in a new age bracket by the same name, and he aims to be highly competitive. He wants to garner his experience from all over the world to not only achieve his goal, but to also *become* his goal. Keep reading to see how he achieves this.

1. What time of day do you run and why?

At one point in life, Jesper dedicated the bulk of his day to serious training. Many of his decisions were made based on what was best overall for his running, and he was eager to travel great distances to incorporate new ideas and experiences into his training. Currently, he faces a three-way battle fought out by time-consuming training goals, real-life work and family demands, and an ideal world where all factors could be balanced.

"There is a gap between what I prefer to do, and what I actually can realize at the moment. My situation has changed in recent years because of full-time work and having three kids." Jesper notes that for an elite runner if the focus on training shifts and other demands compete with the time that was previously allotted to running, it is generally perceived as negative for performance.

He is able to avoid this and achieve a nice balance because his job as a teacher allows him to have a break and incorporate a mid-morning run into his workday. Typically, he'll add in a complementary pre-dawn run before work as well, and if something prevents him from getting out during his workday, he still has the opportunity to get in a late-night workout after 9:00 p.m. The fact that it stays light until very late in the summer months in Scandinavian countries adds bonus hours to evening training! In this way, Jesper can be systematic yet flexible.

Boston Marathon winner Yuki Kawauchi is perhaps the most famous example of this "citizen runner" model. This paradigm, which is also Yuki's nickname, involves the idea that it is in fact beneficial for elite runners to lead busy double lives outside of training, keep a day job and meld into the mold of an ordinary citizen. That is until race day when they reveal an elite singlet under their business attire and whiz by the professional athletes that spend their days on a train-race-repeat mode with little margin for anything else.

This can lead to situations that professional runners

don't have to think about, such as this anecdote after Yuki's historic win: "Sorry, but I won the Boston Marathon," Yuki said to his boss back in his native Japan shortly after his win. "Is it possible to have another day off?" Yet some say that having other significant things to focus on, such as a job or a family, is a benefit rather than an obstacle as it can reduce burnout in a training cycle.

***

"Sorry, but I won the Boston Marathon, is it possible to have another day off?"

–Citizen Runner Yuki Kawauchi, who holds down a full-time job while winning marathons worldwide. (As quoted by the New York Times)

***

2. What do you typically eat before or after training sessions?

During his training, Jesper avoids eating and prefers to pay close attention to his fluid uptake, which he feels is an essential component while running long distances. He will have a snack before running, such as a banana, white bread, or an energy bar, and he enjoys a Coca-Cola with some rye bread after.

As part of his training diet, Jesper shares that he uses "a low residue diet, which features a lot of carbs but no fiber. This way, you benefit from a great deal of energy without having a lot of fiber that fills up your stomach. You can get energized and feel a bit lighter." This is the reasoning behind eating the rye bread specifically after his running. Rye bread is rich in fiber, which Jesper avoids before a run.

3. What is your special, secret training tip?

Jesper's tip involves "mileage, and the key thing about mileage is to do the tough long runs at a very specific pace before the marathon."

4. Is there any cultural influence, or something going on in your personal life, that impacts your training?

Jesper's life circumstances, namely his full-time job and family, shape his training the most. He says that these factors have limited the freedom he used to have to race and train abroad, but he has embraced his new life and works to find ways to train effectively while staying at home in Denmark.

5. Do you add any other exercise to your marathon preparation for cross training?

Jesper integrates weightlifting into his marathon training. He has discovered that increasing his strength has reduced the post-running soreness he used to suffer from, especially in his tendons. Additionally, he believes it to be effective for injury prevention.

If he does suffer an injury, Jesper substitutes running with training sessions on an elliptical cross trainer. The gliding motion used on a cross trainer is low impact yet still makes for a high-cardio workout. Arm work can be added by focusing on alternating pushing and then pulling the bars. This is typically a bonus for runners that often neglect upper body workouts. Even when Jesper is not injured, he likes to use the elliptical cross trainer to warm up before a treadmill workout session.

6. How long is your marathon training cycle?

Jesper believes that all his training done throughout the year lays the foundation for the marathon. He also shares that he turns to a specific system called the periodization system, which is touted by famed Italian coach Renato Canova, in the weeks leading up to the 26point2. At the start of the periodization system, the focus is on adding speed to your workouts. The closer you get to the marathon date, the more the method includes long runs at specific paces. The underlying idea builds on the speed foundation by adhering to a desired pace until that same pace can be maintained for the duration of the race.

7. What do you eat for breakfast on the day of your marathon?

As noted, before racing Jesper opts for high-carb options, but they must also be low in fiber.

8. What did you eat and drink during the race? At what intervals?

Jesper alternates between using rehydration tablets (he is partial to the High5 brand) and salt tabs that have added caffeine for an additional energy boost.

9. Deep thoughts: what was your mental preparation and focus throughout training and on race day? Do you use any outside running "distractions" (such as music, podcasts, running apps, etc.) while running?

When Jesper is running outdoors, he feels that, "Music distracts me from the beautiful surroundings." He prefers to lose himself in Denmark's wide variety of impressive and often rugged scenery, or in the energy of the crowd on race day.

10. What does your post-race period look like, both for recovery and celebrating? (Note: The celebration after crossing the finish line can serve as motivation that gets you through training and the race!)

"I would like a massage after a race. However, when you have a family it is difficult to have time for everything. But I still would recommend massage!"

Bonus Question: What should you NOT have done in your 26point2?

"Retrospective enlightenment would say training is not a competition. If you train hard, you get better...but it is also crucial to listen to your body and ease up during periods of competition."

Having run the streets of so many countries, Jesper recalled some of his international experiences: "For example, at the European championship the Italian runners ran with white caps, and at specific water stations they threw their caps to the helpers to put ice cubes inside them. The runners took back the caps to cool down. I wish that I would've learned that strategy before taking on the cruel heat in Barcelona in August. You really can learn something new at any point."

Jesper went on to talk about the New York City Marathon. "It was a great experience. The support from the spectators along the course was unbelievable…In a few years from now, I will be a Master runner, and I hope to race in other US city marathons and win this division."

Circling back to Jesper's idea that you become what you do, Jesper anticipates becoming a Master. While he is referring to the race category, based on how he has mastered marathon training to make it compatible with his lifestyle, he will undoubtedly become what he does.

Jesper is always interested in connecting with international racing organizations for collaborative initiatives and elite racing experiences. He is open to representing Denmark in races and may be contacted via his Jesper Faurschou Instagram page.

***

Jesper F., from Denmark, has run in Denmark, Belgium, Brazil, Bulgaria, Croatia, the Czech Republic, Egypt, Finland, France, Germany, Greece, Hungary, Iceland, Ireland, Italy, the Netherlands, Norway, Poland, Portugal, Serbia, Slovakia, Slovenia, South Korea, Spain, Sweden, Switzerland, Thailand, Turkey, Uganda, the UK (where he ran the 26point2 in the London Olympics!), and USA

Mile 11: A Warm Up Good Enough for a Living Legend

Julio M.C. from Spain

Among all the incredibly inspiring international marathon runners I have been fortunate enough to encounter while researching this book and running abroad, I consider Julio M.C. from Spain to deserve the "living legend" distinction. This is not just due to his near-victory on a quest to finish 100 marathons (he currently has 98 under his belt!), his "confession" that he has never suffered an injury in his 35 years as a runner, or his numerous running victories and international experiences, all of which could create fascinating content for another book altogether. All this greatness aside, what classifies Julio as a living legend to me is that he is genuinely charismatic and approachable. The talent, dedication, and passion that he holds for all things running-related is admirable.

This is a marathoner that radiates joy, has a bright smile for all, and is known to dole out positive encouragement to push you on if you happen to come across him at any point of a race. He will also gladly take the time to have a post-run beer and conversation with anyone who wants to know how he has gotten marathon running down to a precise formula that yields excellent results. This open, sincere, and friendly approach makes Julio a standout

Marathon running has led Julio to travel across continents and interact with others who share his passion. Some of his most notable experiences have been in Africa with Ethiopian runners through an organization based out of Spain called "Runners for Ethiopia" (www.runnersforethiopia.com). The mission of this group is to connect runners, coaches, physical therapists, and volunteers that for the most part come from Europe, with the Ethiopian running community for a cultural, athletic and skills exchange. The visitors to Ethiopia benefit greatly while training with local runners and learning techniques in a setting that Julio describes as a "paradise for runners." They also aim to improve the living and training conditions of their hosts through donations of athletic gear and medical supplies. Visiting licensed therapists donate training sessions to Ethiopian physical therapists and focus on how to treat runners. It's a beautiful and successful initiative that culminates in the participation in the Hawassa Marathon near Addis Ababa.

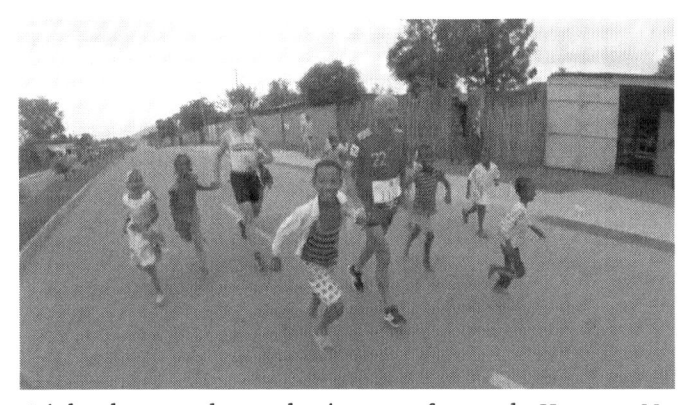

It's hard to say who was having more fun at the Hawassa Marathon in Ethiopia, Julio or the local kids (Photo courtesy of Julio M.C.)

Something distinct to the Ethiopian running style is the way that many warm up before a running workout. Julio is so passionate about these techniques that he enthusiastically shares videos in which he replicates them. He claims that, "These exercises improve both running technique and stride efficiency. Doing these two things properly allows for better running with less effort and will prevent injuries that stem from improper form."

I have seen the videos and tried out the moves myself; they are simple, effective, and addictively FUN!!! Once you see Julio doing the warm-up routine with ease and joy in his videos, you immediately want to try it out yourself. For me, this led to multiple arm whacks on furniture as I mimicked his moves in the limited space of my living room. However, when done outdoors or in a more spacious area, they are a way to add a smile to your workout and start off running with a light step.

According to Julio, almost all of the runners in Meskel Square employ the same warm-up practice. This square is the nucleus of running in Addis Ababa, and those who train there follow in the footsteps of greats such as Haile Gebrselassie and Abebe Bikila. In smaller towns throughout Ethiopia, I've seen similar central squares where runners hang out and work out, and the atmosphere always looks spirited.

Julio is a gem of a person and was willing to go into great depth on many topics featured in this book, and freely share his distinctive insight. Let's keep Julio, his attitude, and his training style in mind as he approaches becoming a 100-time marathoner!

1. What time of day do you run and why?

Julio prefers morning training sessions. "Your mind and body are more relaxed in the morning and less influenced by problems, worries, or pending tasks." He likes the Andalusian sun to be higher in the sky during the winter mornings, so he will hold off until 11:00 a.m. or so before heading out, but in the summer months he has no choice other than to leave earlier to avoid temperatures of up to 115 Fahrenheit (46 Celsius). It's not a humid heat where Julio resides, but it can feel like the depths of an oven from June to September.

2. What do you typically eat before or after training sessions?

Julio partakes in the breakfast most typically seen throughout the region of Andalusia where he lives. It consists of coffee with milk, and toast (in his case, he adds marmalade or honey). Post-run he'll refuel and rehydrate with an isotonic beverage, a banana or apple, and on occasion, a mix of nuts and dried fruit such as walnuts with dates or almonds with figs.

3. What is your special, secret training tip?

"I have no real secrets, but I have to confess I have one unusual quirk. During my 35 years of running, in which my mileage has added up to over two trips around the Earth, I have never suffered an injury! I once had a small muscle strain when running the Boston Marathon, but very soon after I was fine again. My running friends almost all have some recurring injuries they struggle with.

When they ask me what my trick is, I tell them that I simply listen to my body. **Our bodies are constantly sending us signals, and the key is to learn how to interpret them**. Sometimes you face a tougher workout that you don't feel like doing. In those cases, I advise replacing it with something light, because your body is warning you that on that specific day it could be prone to injury." When you treat your body kindly, an invitation to successful results is extended.

Julio also feels that the beloved warm-up routine he learned in Ethiopia helps him avoid injury. "It takes only about ten minutes, but it prepares you in a really important way for the exercise you're about to do." He also dedicates about five minutes of time to focus on stretching after he cools down. He believes that regularly doing both of these things allows him to feel great after his workouts and races.

4. Is there any cultural influence, or something going on in your personal life, that impacts your training?

At one point, due to life circumstances, including the arrival of twin baby boys, Julio had to give up his ideal running times completely. In doing so, he was often out running at times when the majority of people he'd encounter were on their way to the next *discoteca* to finish off their night out. It was around this time that Julio developed a standard response to a comment he often fielded from people that said they too would like to train as he does, but simply lacked the time. Julio's steadfast reply was that for the pursuit of a real passion, you can always shave off a bit of time from your sleep and diversion, and dedicate that to your running goal.

Julio also equates his running to an "escape valve for high stress," namely from work-related issues. Well said! I have trained for years along the same picturesque routes that Julio runs in Andalusia, and I can also confirm that any stress will leave your mind, if only for a moment, when you are faced with a spectacular sunrise emerging over those particular landscapes.

5. Do you add any other exercise to your marathon preparation for cross training?

Julio finds it useful to incorporate swimming into his training program. He aims for two or three pool sessions a week in which he looks to tone his upper-body muscles while in the water.

Swimming also benefits tired and well-worked legs. While not an official stroke for competitive swimming, **after a long run, the sidestroke is especially restorative**. This is because it provides a smooth, flowing movement that alleviates tightness in the legs and hips. This stroke involves lying on your side and kicking your legs like scissors, much like a lifeguard would if he or she was towing a swimmer back to shore. The motion serves to loosen the hip area, which is notorious for being tight. Since your head is out of the water, it's not necessary to time the breathing, and many find that relaxing as well.

6. How long is your marathon training cycle?

"Since I usually do about six to seven marathons a year, I'm basically training year-round, although I usually take a full week off from running after each marathon."

7. What do you eat for breakfast on the day of your marathon?

Julio maintains his simple breakfast toast with jam or

honey and a cup of coffee on race day. He also points out that he's shocked when he travels to a marathon destination and notices at the hotel breakfast what he considers to be an excessive amount of food that some marathoners eat on race day. He believes that fueling done in the week leading up to the race is what has the most impact and that the race day meal shouldn't be too big.

8. What did you eat and drink during the race? At what intervals?

Julio also feels that due to his extensive experience, his need to refuel and rehydrate during his 26point2 is considerably reduced. His body has simply adapted to the distance over time and he finds drinking anything beyond water to be excessive. He doesn't even feel a great need to stop for water unless it's very hot out. "I should actually get a discount on the marathon registration fees because I hardly touch anything set out at the aid stations," he says with a laugh.

He is quick to state in his light-hearted and easy way that each runner has a unique path and that just because this strategy works for him doesn't mean that it is ideal for everyone.

9. Deep thoughts: what was your mental preparation and focus throughout training and on race day? Do you use any outside running "distractions" (such as music, podcasts, running apps, etc.) while running?

"My strategy is to frame the first half of the race as a time to rest and relax. You won't have any problems during that part if you've trained. After you pass the 25 km mark (15.5 miles) and your legs start to feel heavy, you can start to count the kilometers that you have left and compare them with those of your well-known training routes."

Since Julio has so much experience, he instinctively knows how his pacing will translate into a finishing time. If he's struggling with his speed in a race, he'll do the math in his head and come up with a compromise of split times that allows him to reduce his pace a bit yet still achieve a finishing time that he feels good about.

Julio enjoys listening to music while running, but will forgo the headphones when running with others, as the priority for him is to enjoy the company of fellow runners. He also logs his running data on the Strava app, since this allows him to be part of a virtual running community that shares stories and supports its members.

10. What does your post-race period look like, both for recovery and celebrating? (Note: The celebration after crossing the finish line can serve as motivation that gets you through training and the race!)

Since Julio is such a social person, it makes perfect sense that one of the parts he loves most about the post-race experience is recounting the impressions he got from each kilometer with his running community online. He looks forward to updating his blog, www.juliomolinacastellano.blogpost.com, with descriptions, photos, and marathon videos. How Julio achieves his remarkable times while documenting his races with pictures and videos is beyond me, but he feels, "These are great souvenirs of each race experience and I have a ton of fun making them."

Perhaps since Julio limits his consumption of fluid in his 26point2, he feels incredibly thirsty after he crosses the finish line and claims that the best way to solve this issue is to visit the beer truck. "I consume all of the beer that I can, and if it's with my running friends, that's even better."

Bonus Question: What should you NOT have done in your 26point2?

Julio advises marathoners not to forget that painful chafing is a distinct possibility during the race. To avoid this, he protects delicate areas that are prone to chafing with special moisture absorbing patches. The Compeed brand (www.compeed.com) is his favorite. He will also **coat his feet and inner-**

thigh area with petroleum jelly. "It's strange to me to see people bleeding in very sensitive areas during races because the steps needed to avoid chafing are really quite simple."

With this last comment, Julio encompasses why his expertise gathered over 35 years of running is so valuable. What seems like simple common sense to him could be a brand-new idea that could make or break the racing experience of a newer runner. Spanish speaking runners have the opportunity to benefit directly from Julio's advice, and training plans through his *Injerateams* initiative.

In a nod to the spongy, bread-like base of the Ethiopian diet called *injera*, Julio named the training group he leads *Injerateams*. He is aware that numerous training groups already exist, so he created a fresh training perspective to contribute something different yet effective. Julio brought back a lot of knowledge from Ethiopia that impacted his running greatly and readily shares it through his training group.

Through *Injerateams*, Julio and other coaches collaborate to provide a range of personalized training components, including marathon coaching; goal setting activities; psychological support for motivation and pre-race anxiety; and valuable information infused with training tips from Ethiopia. For anyone that wants to up their running IQ with the helpful information that Julio facilitates through this supportive community, find out more at www.injerateams.com (all information is in Spanish). The rest of us can await news of Julio's successful 100th marathon. People from around the world will be raising a beer to this remarkable achievement. *Salud* Julio!

***

Julio M.C., from Spain, has run in Spain, Ethiopia, Germany, Ireland, Italy, the Netherlands, Switzerland, the UK, and USA

Mile 12: Farm to Fork Training

Alastair N. from South Africa

What do a plant-based diet grown right at home and a new yoga practice have to do with marathon training? For South African marathoner Alastair N., these serve as the basis of both his training and his lifestyle. The time leading up to Al's marathon coincided with many transitions in his life, a major one being a move from the busy and at times chaotic capital city of Maputo, Mozambique, to the quiet mountain village where he currently resides in South Africa. The relocation from an urban setting to rural life came hand-in-hand with a lifestyle overhaul that focused on becoming vegetarian. Al and his family found it easier to make this shift in their new environment due to the availability of fresh seasonal produce, which was locally sourced.

He also determined that yoga was highly beneficial to his training plan and now has plans to make it a more central component of the preparation for his next marathon. These two additions help him to feel better equipped to take on his 26point2. Below he shares exactly why.

1. What time of day do you run and why?

I'm sure that there is a marathoner out there that has exclusively trained on an indoor treadmill, but I have yet to encounter that person. Most runners are at the mercy of the weather. Al seasonally tweaks his training in this regard. "In winter here, (as it was when training for the Cape Town Marathon that I ran in September) I run in the evenings after work during weekdays, sometimes at night around 9:00–10:00 p.m.

This was just because I don't enjoy getting up and running the cold mornings and then going to work. Now in summer, I am running in early mornings as it gets light at 4:45–5:00 a.m. and this is lovely." **Making seasonal shifts to your running schedule can help you to enjoy the highlights of the different times of year** while reducing the impacts of less-than-desirable conditions.

2. What do you typically eat before or after training sessions?

The change that Al and his family made in their lifestyle choices when they moved to a more rural area led them to fully embrace a "farm-to-fork" approach to eating and control their food sourcing more closely. They committed to eating a mostly plant-based diet, but they decided to allow for one major exception: eggs. The family adds eggs to their meals to provide a complete protein and makes it a point to source their eggs from local chickens that roam their neighbors' fields.

There is a big learning curve involved with the shift to this diet, especially while training for a marathon. It requires a lot of trial and error to achieve the right balance of nutrients for optimal fueling. Al found ways to make it possible to meet his amplified nutritional needs while training even while adopting a mostly vegan approach. He added extra protein in the morning by sprinkling chia seeds on everything he ate at breakfast, and at lunch he paired his dishes with a healthy portion of creamy hummus. The local eggs he ate were also on regular rotation. "Before a long run, I eat one or two bananas and a tomato omelet. After the run, I have another plant-protein mix and another omelet and more fruit."

Scott Jurek, a US-based runner and author who has won nearly all of the elite races in the ultra-running sector, also adheres to a vegetarian diet (in his case strictly vegan). He claims this lifestyle choice is the cornerstone of the foundation of his extraordinary success. Scott defies the idea that you can't fuel for long-distance endeavors while eating a vegan diet, and his victories and record-setting times in prestigious 100-mile races validate his nutritional choices.

Scott promotes the abundant consumption of salads, homemade smoothies, and buckwheat pancakes among the many other ideas that are found in his bestselling book, *Eat and Run* (available at www.scottjurek.com). Scott has ideas for grab-and-go vegan options while training or for fueling during a race, including rice and bean burritos, hummus with olives in tortilla wraps, and bread with quinoa spread. Scott finds he gets positive results when he avoids highly processed food, and Al also subscribes to this idea.

3. What is your special, secret training tip?

Al's top tip is to invest some real time in researching various training plans to find the one best suited to the race, your personal goals, and the surrounding circumstances. "I found one that worked for me and just stuck to it," he says.

4. Is there any cultural influence, or something going on in your personal life, that impacts your training?

Al faced significant life changes amid his marathon preparation but decided to use his training sessions as an escape from the stress he was facing. In doing so, he was able to bolster his mental wellbeing throughout the transitions. Life was especially hectic during this time, as he had an international move, committed to his new diet and lifestyle, and started up his own company, just as his training level was picking up. He said that these personal circumstances made it extremely challenging to find time to train, "but at the same time, the running was very therapeutic, and it was so great to have a goal."

5. Do you add any other exercise to your marathon preparation for cross training?

"I stretched every day and did yoga as cross training." It is decidedly beneficial for runners to incorporate yoga into their training. A consistent practice leads to increased flexibility and strength, and also contributes to improved respiration, energy, and vitality. Yoga routines vary, but those involving a series of fluid postures can stretch out tight areas in the body that are prone to the stiffness brought on by the mechanics of running. A yoga practice can be done almost anywhere, even with no equipment. An array of yoga classes specifically geared towards runners is also available.

I turn to a yoga series created by a marathoner named Rebecca Pacheco. Rebecca sees the practice through the lens of a runner and as a result, her YouTube yoga tutorials intuitively know how to unlock intense muscle tension that runners can experience. I cannot overstate the benefits I've seen when adding her postures to my running repertoire. Her approach makes running and yoga feel intrinsically connected. To learn more about this inspirational yogi marathoner see www.rebeccapacheco.com.

6. How long is your marathon training cycle?

"Fifteen weeks. Circumstance really brought that on, with the move, etc. I found a program for that length of time, and it turned out to be enough."

7. What do you eat for breakfast on the day of your marathon?

"Two bananas and a tomato omelet with three eggs no coincidence that Al's race day meal was identical to h' diet. It's deeply reported that consistency is critical fr sults on race day.

8. What did you eat and drink during the intervals?

"I ran with a rehydration pack with) it. I had used it on all my long training r Cape Town was in a water crisis and I d to it. I also wanted to reduce my usr

CPT Marathon was very well prepared. They had water sachets available at specific places, roughly every 3–5 km (1.5–3 miles). I also ran with GU gels. I take one every 45 minutes for energy." Hopefully, Al's Earth-friendly marathon approach will become the norm, and innovative solutions will help manage the waste and plastic use that marathons generate.

9. Deep thoughts: what was your mental preparation and focus throughout training and on race day? Do you use any outside running "distractions" (such as music, podcasts, running apps, etc.) while running?

"I don't use any music or podcasts etc. unless I run on a treadmill in a hotel when traveling. In some ways, this started as a security thing. I'd go running without anything obvious on me to be less of a target for street crime in Maputo before our move. But I also like it. It's time to be with me and let my thoughts wander. We live in a small village in the mountains, so a lot of my running is trail running or dirt-road running. It's lovely to enjoy the outdoors."

Al lived previously in Maputo, which like many capital cities of Africa, pulses with a frantic energy. It is best to stay fully alert and focused while trying to run in any place with unpredictable traffic or potential personal safety hazards.

During his race in Cape Town, South Africa, Al found that the crowd support "made a massive difference." It was the reason he ran with a smile for most of the race and was able to oak up the energy that radiated off everyone involved. He felt trifecta of pride in his accomplishment, respect for all of his low marathoners out on the course, and a deep appreciation ll the people of Cape Town who turned out to motivate the ers. "It was amazing."

10. What does your post-race period look like, both for re- and celebrating? (Note: The celebration after crossing the ne can serve as motivation that gets you through training ace!)

"My family was there; my girls were five and seven. They loved that their dad had been part of this big, cool event." After the race, the family celebrated with a big vegan meal at a restaurant and enjoyed a relaxing time on the waterfront before Al broke away for an afternoon nap.

Bonus Question: What should you NOT have done in your 26point2?

Here Al circles back to his belief that yoga and running complement each other in a highly beneficial way. He goes on to say that increased running distances should go hand-in-hand with more time dedicated to yoga practice. When he voiced his only regret about his training, he emphatically stated, "I should have done more yoga!"

Al's journey from a well-researched training plan in one country to the finish line in another saw vital changes in his life along the way. He is grateful that the marathon experience formed a part of his transition and tied in with the addition of a healthy diet and yoga practice to his life. Even though the training required considerable commitment during a hectic time, in the end it was a positive learning experience with lasting impacts.

***

Alastair N., from South Africa, has run in South Africa, Mozambique, Uganda, and USA

Mile 13: Run Walk Run and Get the Job Done

Christine D. from USA

US Olympic runner Jeff Galloway promotes the Run-Walk-Run method to achieve outstanding race results with significant injury risk reduction. The main idea of this technique is to add planned walking intervals into a run to avoid fatigue and muscle strain. Runners claim that the popular method helps them to prepare for and take on the marathon physically, but what's interesting about the perspective that runner Christine D. from USA holds is how the Run-Walk-Run method provided her with benefits and support *psychologically*. Especially during a hectic time in life, the method put a refreshing spin on her view of the race and training cycle and contributed to rewarding results.

Christine found herself taking on the challenge of marathon training amidst a particularly busy phase in life. In addition to her running program, she felt like a Cirque de Soleil juggler, keeping the balls of full-time work, graduate school studies, and activities relating to the role of maid of honor (at a destination wedding in Mexico, no less) all afloat. The wedding date was set shortly after her race, which spiked Christine's apprehension about the training plan she needed to complete beforehand.

Christine is one of the most well-studied runners I have ever met: she consults with professional running coaches for her races, thoughtfully evaluates different training plans, and learns all the ins and outs of everything running-related, including stretching, strength training, diet, speed/distance/hill workouts, etc., etc., etc. I could go on and on about the effort Christine puts into her training before she even laces up her shoes! She consistently strives to learn more about running and then puts that knowledge into practice.

In spite of her overloaded schedule during her training for the Marine Corps Marathon in Washington DC, USA, this drive to learn more led Christine to find the time to escape and attend a talk by Jeff Galloway who was discussing the Run-Walk-Run method. She found Jeff to be a highly persuasive speaker as he supported his technique with experiences, testimonials, and — key for Christine's sharp mind — data to back it all up.

Something major clicked with Christine during the presentation, and she felt a shift in her perspective towards the race and the training involved. As she learned more about the Run-Walk-Run approach, she came to see the marathon as something to be enjoyed, not simply "get through." With this new technique, she gave herself permission to relish in the programmed walking breaks instead of pushing through the running and eventually suffering. The walking intervals gave her more time to notice her surroundings, and she now viewed the 26point2 as a block of time to take pleasure in something she loved. In doing so, she was still able to get highly positive results.

As Christine embraced this shift, she realized that her goal of running the 26point2 was manageable, even with all the other commitments she had going on in her life. She happily noted that in addition to providing a mental break, the walking intervals allowed her to savor the race day experience as she felt less tired than she had anticipated throughout the run.

Christine went on to describe that one must employ discipline when doing the walking breaks because early on in the race, adrenaline makes it extremely challenging to slow down. The force and energy of the other runners carry you along, and you feel almost as if you are flying in the beginning. However, if you go out too fast, it is very possible to hit a wall as the race progresses.

The programmed walking breaks change this scenario. By using them early on, later fatigue is diminished. Christine found they also provided a mental boost because knowing that she could take the breaks led her to reframe the whole experience in a more relaxed way.

The questions below provide a detailed view of how Christine approaches running marathons.

1. What time of day do you run and why?

Christine trains as early as possible, although her start times shift throughout the year. She leaves earlier in summer to avoid the heat and later in winter to avoid the dark.

2. What do you typically eat before or after training sessions?

Before any long run, Christine will opt for a banana and half a CLIF bar (Christine's a vegetarian and CLIF bars are a vegan fueling option).

3. What is your special, secret training tip?

"I learned it from Jeff Galloway: You can walk a lot and still get an admirable time in your marathon. Sometimes when I don't want too much wear and tear, I do walk breaks during my long runs, too. This 'jogged' a memory for me…I once passed a teammate who took a walking break during a 5K race in college, and I thought, 'Omg get with the program this is college XC [cross-country running].' And then that runner proceeded to beat me. Unfortunately, it took me many years after that day to accept that walking is a part of running."

***

"Those with the right Run-Walk-Run adjustments are strong to the finish. They are the "passers" not the "passees" during the last few miles which is very empowering."

–Jeff Galloway

***

I recently tried out Christine's approach and can attest to her perspective. I used the method during a marathon with an extreme elevation profile and even so I found that it was indeed a struggle to employ the walking intervals early on. It took discipline to make myself do the breaks when I felt great and didn't want to slow down. Additionally, I was faced with comments such as, "Come on, races are for running not walking!" that some fellow runners shared with me. After the mid-point mark, however, I started feeling grateful for the breaks. I'm happy to share that for the last half hour of the race, I allowed myself to skip the walk breaks altogether. I felt so great that I decided to turn them into sprint breaks! This resulted in negative splits, a fantastic finish, and cheers from those same participants that had previously felt the need to comment on the method I was using. It was ironic that at that point they were out of energy and forced to finish the race at a slow stumble. In addition, my recovery was incredibly fast. After using the Run-Walk-Run method, I felt I could do another 26point2 the very next day! *The Run-Walk-Run Method* book outlines the many ways that these strategies can give you a new lease on your marathon life. More information can be found at Jeff Galloway's website: www.jeffgalloway.com.

4. Is there any cultural influence, or something going on in your personal life, that impacts your training?

"One thing that always puts an extra pep in my step is the Boston Marathon. The days and weeks immediately afterward fill me with motivation. Last year, the sub-two-hour marathon attempt really motivated me, and still to this day, I think about what goes on in those professional runners' heads while I'm focused on just trying to keep a certain pace in a race." For Christine, Boston's Marathon Monday is a holiday, and for her the celebration continues long past the race and inspires her running for months to come.

5. Do you add any other exercise to your marathon preparation for cross training?

Christine adds in strength training in a unique way. In addition to her (well-planned and faithfully executed) endurance building, she incorporates mini squat sessions throughout the day; even when at work. She might do a quick set of clandestine squats in the ladies' room and feels that even smaller efforts add up to significant benefits. She adds in other active moments, such as taking the stairs and doing lunchtime walks or yoga sessions, that both clear her mind and boost her energy. Christine is at the same time a dedicated runner and a dedicated professional that finds ways to link the two.

6. How long is your marathon training cycle?

Christine is very active and says, "I usually have a decent base just about any time of the year." As such, she can get prepared for a marathon within 15 weeks.

7. What do you eat for breakfast on the day of your marathon?

Ironically, part of this intelligent runner's race day breakfast is the taffy-like American candy called Airheads! She appreciates the boost of sheer energy that they give her. Additionally, before any race she will consume one GU energy gel followed by water.

8. What did you eat and drink during the race? At what intervals?

During a marathon, Christine relies on water and takes a GU gel every 5 miles (8 km).

9. Deep thoughts: what was your mental preparation and focus throughout training and on race day? Do you use any outside running "distractions" (such as music, podcasts, running apps, etc.) while running?

"I tell myself something like 'see you on the other side' as if post-race Christine is a different person from pre-race Christine."

I love this psychological construct! Aren't all runners somehow transformed post-race regardless of the outcome? Each race is a learning experience. We get to know more not only about the practical details of what works for our racing, but also about ourselves.

10. What does your post-race period look like, both for recovery and celebrating? (Note: The celebration after crossing the finish line can serve as motivation that gets you through training and the race!)

"If there's a beer in sight after crossing the finish line, I will most definitely drink it. That's about it. I'll have a few easy days after a hard effort and a few more alcoholic beverages." Cheers to a job well done!

Bonus Question: What should you NOT have done in your 26point2?

Christine strongly advises against stopping movement after crossing the finish line of a marathon. "Walk, walk, walk. Use the foam roller if there's one at the medical tent. Walk back to your hotel room or apartment if possible. Walk that evening before going to bed. I made the huge mistake of crossing the line of my first marathon, patting myself on the back, and then sitting for about an hour, talking with friends. Afterward, I couldn't move normally for days."

When Christine shifted her perception about taking walking breaks while training and racing, magic ensued. The belief that strong runners don't implement walking breaks is simply untrue. The entire marathon experience, including the training cycle, can be more manageable and indeed enjoyable when walking breaks are used. They can even greatly enhance your results!

Jeff Galloway further motivates runners by stating, "To reach the finish line in a marathon is to enter an elite group: only about one-tenth of one percent of the population does it." Christine is part of this group already, and it is clear that with her focused, driven, and intelligent marathon preparation she will soon be living her dream and running the streets of Boston among the greats. Christine, I will be the first to cheer you on during Marathon Monday, especially during your walk breaks. Brava!

***

Christine D., from USA, has run in USA, Austria, Argentina, Belgium, the Czech Republic, Denmark, Germany, Ireland, Italy, the Netherlands, Switzerland, and the UK

Mile 14: I Carried It, or Perhaps It Carried me, to the Finish Line

Togz T. from the Philippines

Togz T. is originally from the Philippines and has international marathon racing experience ranging from such far-flung places as Thailand, Greece, and Germany. His quirky approach to long distance running, and indeed to certain aspects of life in general, always prevails. Togz embraces different aspects of the sport with genuine enthusiasm and finds joy in the small details of running as he forges an innovative path to reach his goals.

Imagine a person who thrives on marching to the beat of his own drum, someone who insists on writing "wordz" that end with -s with a -z. Togz refuses to mold to the conventional, and that spirit is found in his training as well.

Togz also makes a point to find a positive balance between his dedicated training plan and his role as a father. In order to meet his family's childcare and household needs, Togz dramatically alters his training schedule and on most occasions finds himself heading out to get a run in when most of us are either deep in dreamland or returning home from a festive night out.

When traveling for marathons, Togz embraces the local customs. He possesses a sincere appreciation for the smaller details found in the racing experience, taking note of the cheerful and supportive volunteers at aid stations, the high-fives from kids and adults, and the jubilant energy given off by marathon onlookers.

Most notably, Togz reveled in the history, lore, and culture surrounding the Athens Marathon in Greece (or as two Greek marathon-running brothers I know call it, "The Original"). Togz shared that he "had the opportunity to trace the footsteps of Pheidippides from Marathon to Athens," and states with a bit of wry humor, "and I survived." He credits this in part to the kindness of the fans that lined up to support the runners.

This landmark racecourse was a dream for Togz, and the original roots of the modern marathon merit a bit of description. The route is said to roughly follow the path that Pheidippides, a messenger from Athens, ran to share the news of a victory in battle with the Persians. Legend has it that after proclaiming *"Nike! Nike! Nenikikamen"* (Victory! Victory! Rejoice, we conquer!) he collapsed and promptly died.

In previous travels to Greece, I have been lucky enough to explore the original marathon route, albeit by car, and I can fully appreciate the magnetic draw Togz felt to the race; the route is nothing short of inspiring. Runners start off from the town of Marathon (where the 26point2 gets its name) in eastern Greece and make a special loop to observe a battleground site and monument to Athenian soldiers that fought for democracy. They then carry on through rolling farmland and a smattering of villages until they reach the outskirts of the great metropolis of Athens.

Upon reaching the city, another runner greets the racers. Dromeas is the name of a two-story tall modern sculpture of a marathoner made of stacks upon stacks of sheets of glass. The overall effect embodies the feeling of a runner in windswept motion. However, the contemporary feel of the sculpture dramatically contrasts with the ancient structures towering over the racecourse.

The magnificent complex of the Acropolis citadel peers down on runners from its lofty position and the race features a spectacular finish in the Olympic stadium which hosted the 1896 Olympics and is the birthplace of the modern games. Some Athens-based race organizations present marathon finishers with small ceramic vases, in a nod to what the historic first Olympic Games provided as "race swag."

The story of Pheidippides' fated run might be historical lore and not entirely correct, but the approximate distance and route are celebrated and carry on today in the modern marathon. Comparisons have been made that a runner running the marathon in Athens is akin to a golfer playing on the original golf course of St. Andrews in Scotland, thought to be the cradle of the game. Others have gone so far as to classify the renowned Athens marathon experience as a pilgrimage of sorts to the "Cathedral of Running." Togz feels fortunate not only to have run this racecourse steeped in history but also for the gestures of the fans that lined the route. He fondly recalls an olive branch offered up by a small boy.

Thought to symbolize glory in former times, the olive branch is still symbolic today. The tradition of locals handing them out to encourage the runners stems from the ancient Olympic Games where the winners were crowned with twisted olive branches. Togz felt that the gesture transcended time, language, and culture and clung to the branch for the remainder of his race. The impact the boy's gesture had on him was clear: "I carried it, or perhaps it carried me, until the finish line."

With added "tipz" and interesting "momentz," Togz shares his marathon chronicles and his outlook on the sport, all with his signature twist.

1. What time of day do you run and why?

Togz is no sloth. He will do whatever it takes to get in a workout during his marathon training, even if that means defying norms and standards and discovering ways to get in a run in any way possible, at any time possible. This point is proven by his pre-dawn (extremely pre-dawn) departures from his house in order to get in solid, long-distance workouts while allowing him to return home by 5:30 or 6:00 a.m.

For Togz, it is not uncommon to begin a standard weekday run between 3:00 and 4:00 a.m. (for a duration of one to two hours). He'll tackle his weekend long runs as early as 2:30 a.m. (for a run around three hours). He justifies this unconventional option because the way he sees it, "Itz the free time I choose so I can still help out with my household and with the kidz."

2. What do you typically eat before or after training sessions?

Togz is used to running on an empty stomach, perhaps as a result of starting out so early. However, as a marathon date approaches, he starts using gels taken with water for his longer runs so that his body adapts to them for the race. That way, on marathon day there are no surprises. He also makes it a habit to eat a lot of pasta during his training cycle.

3. What is your special, secret training tip?

"I would say that you just have to enjoy it (most of the time), and the rest will follow!" With his customary enthusiasm, many emojis were added here to drive home Togz's point. :) :) :)

4. Is there any cultural influence, or something going on in your personal life, that impacts your training?

As Togz has such a distinct vision of what his training looks like, he says that cultural factors don't really influence him.

5. Do you add any other exercise to your marathon preparation for cross training?

Togz incorporates basic stretching to his post-run routine and will often do planks and sit-ups for additional core strength. Core strength is a key component to proper running form. The more strength you have in the trunk, the easier it is to maintain an efficient and upright posture. A weaker core makes it more difficult to keep up good posture deep into a long run and energy (mental and physical) that is needed to cover the remaining distance is expended on maintaining the correct form. However, if the core is strong, the proper running form should prevail.

When done correctly, planks contribute to strengthening the core, and they also offer an added advantage of simultaneously working other muscle groups such as those in the arms and shoulders. These are areas that are often overlooked by runners, so planks contribute to full-body strengthening. They also encourage balance and even stretch out areas that are notoriously tight for runners, including the hamstrings, the arches of the feet and even the hardworking toes.

Planks can be done just about anywhere. I can be found doing planks in the kitchen while I'm waiting for the water for my tea to boil; while playing at the beach or on the playground with my kiddo; and while waiting for my dog to endlessly sniff every tree and shrub in her immediate area while on a walk in the park. I even know of office teams that do plank challenges at work. The fact that they can be done in a minimal timeframe and require no change in wardrobe makes them easy to do, even while dressed in professional attire.

6. How long is your marathon training cycle?

Togz typically maintains a solid running base, and for his marathons he allots 12 weeks to a focused training cycle.

7. What do you eat for breakfast on the day of your marathon?

Togz has a generous and balanced breakfast in which macronutrients play a big role, and he also insists upon starting his hydration well before the pistol sounds at the start of the race. "I usually have coffee, eggs, toast with butter, and a small serving of pasta three hours before the race. Itz one of my usual breakfasts and the pasta is often a leftover from dinner. Plenty of water, but thatz usual."

8. What did you eat and drink during the race? At what intervals?

During the 26point2, Togz distributes his hydration and fueling into small, manageable portions. He aims to take just two sips of water at each aid station from start to finish. At the halfway point, he'll start taking gels at 30-minute intervals. His notion is that during the first portion of his race, his body is still drawing on his big breakfast, but during the second part he begins to lose steam and can use the gels for fuel as he increases his effort to reach the finish line.

9. Deep thoughts: what was your mental preparation and focus throughout training and on race day? Do you use any outside running "distractions" (such as music, podcasts, running apps, etc.) while running?

"In preparing for a marathon, I have a goal in mind and a plan (written, but still flexible). I usually consult with friends that have had success in running." Throughout his training cycle, Togz periodically pulls out this plan to review his progress, troubleshoot where he sees any potential difficulties or gaps in his training, and to celebrate small victories made along the way. **Getting your training plan in writing binds you more tightly to it and serves as a tangible reference.**

10. What does your post-race period look like, both for recovery and celebrating? (Note: The celebration after crossing the finish line can serve as motivation that gets you through training and the race!)

Togz has a very clear post-race priority: "The beer!" He goes on to say that that's not in fact his only focus, and he also enjoys a celebratory meal with family and looks forward to getting to bed that night. He realized the great importance of rest and recovery but shares that, "Sometimes I am also too tired to sleep!"

Many over-exhausted marathon runners report that it's

hard to immediately unwind after the big race. The hybrid feeling of being exhausted and exhilarated after completing a 26point2 is familiar to many, but sleep eventually comes. The important thing is to try and let your body relax. I can only imagine that this mix of emotions is heightened after running in such an emblematic race as the Athens Marathon.

Togz has a personality that lends to an open, easy approach to running. Due to his expat background and international running experiences, he has even been named a marathon international ambassador at the Vienna City Marathon and embraces the opportunity to meet and exchange experiences with runners from all over the world. "Good timez" and meaningful connections with others accompany him whenever he races, so I can't imagine a more perfect person to engage with runners while representing his home country.

***

Togz T., from the Philippines, has run in Austria, Greece, and Thailand

Mile 15: I Get by With a Little Help from My Fans
Sarah R. from the UK

British runner Sarah R.'s enthusiasm for sharing her marathon experience is on par with her energetic zombie-slaying running workouts. Luckily for us, Sarah is a dynamic storyteller who treated all aspects of her marathon as a wide-open book. She was happy to go into detail about the various emotional and physical components that were part of her challenge when it came to running a marathon, and her story is incredibly uplifting.

Without question, what stood out for Sarah during her 26point2 were the energetic and frenzied crowds and the general support and admiration for runners that overflowed from the community that day. Sarah described this as an incredible sensation that can be felt throughout the entire body, and apparently this is common for many racers to experience while running in the UK. The UK has a history of highly successful marathoners, the London Marathon is one of the most iconic in the world, and the fan base for runners all over the country is nothing short of extraordinary.

From the very young to the very old, locals come out to support marathoners and make it a point to have a great time while doing so. The impact of their joyous presence can't be ignored. For example, the London Marathon is often referred to as a 26point2 mile long-block party. It is also said that many pubs enjoy their biggest business days of the year if the marathon route passes by. It's hard to imagine something more festive.

While not a groundbreaking concept, on race day Sarah

decided to put her first name on the front of her shirt, and in the context of her British marathon, she was exceedingly glad she did. As she ran past the crowds, the spectators cheered her on by name. Sarah felt that the personalized support gave a huge and continuous energy boost.

It is also tradition that the crowds at races in the UK come prepared with little treats to give out to the runners as they pass by. This practice is so typical that now some runners count on it and don't bring as many of their own energy boosters. In Sarah's case, the fan-provided treat came in the form of a gummy candy called Jelly Babies.

Jelly Babies are brightly colored sweets from England in the form of...well, chubby babies. They are so funny-looking that I laughed out loud when I first saw them. They are sweet, have just the right amount of chew, and provide a quick zap of energy. Fun fact: at the end of World War II the name of this British candy briefly was changed to Peace Babies to mark the end of the fighting. Jelly Babies have a marked history in the country and are very much a nostalgic and recognized candy. Sarah says, "I munched on tons of Jelly Babies that the crowds handed out to the runners...There were kids as young as five giving me Jelly Babies and high fives. Brilliant!"

As far as her marathon training, Sarah was doing that delicate dance familiar to many, which involves the complexities and time restraints found when mixing marathon training, working full time and raising small children. One interesting way she got around this was by tweaking a common practice that many runners report using.

The majority of the runners that I've spoken with share that they save the long runs for Sundays. This practice holds true even more so for the working parent contingency. However, Sarah discovered that in her case, using the weekend for a long run proved to be more exhausting than beneficial. "The further into my training I got, the more I realized I desperately needed the recovery time (which meant being kid-free for a couple of hours so that I could relax). So, I decided that it was more convenient to take a day off work as annual leave on the days that I had to run more than 18 miles. This allowed me to have a bath and relax before I would pick the kids up from kindergarten." To borrow Sarah's phrase, brilliant! The long runs can of course be done on Sundays, but for parents, as Sarah rightfully points out, the idea of any recovery time afterward when there are little ones around with varying needs (and demands ;)) is a legitimate challenge that needs to be taken into consideration.

As I was training for a 26point2 for the first time since I had changed my status to "marathon mama," the longest and hardest run of my training fell on my baby's first birthday. I got up extremely early to complete my 3+ hour route and was back just as my little family was waking up to enjoy the day of celebrating.

While there is no doubt in my mind that it was a fun and special day for all of us, around 4:00 p.m. that afternoon, I felt a considerable dip in energy. We were at the zoo, the crowds of small kids were chaotic, and I was pushing the stroller about in the hot sun. I felt exhausted and should have employed a bit of rest and recovery after my long workout, as opposed to diving into a busy day head-on.

What I did not consider at the time was what the aftermath that the lack of rest after my long haul entailed. Spending some of that day relaxing would have been beneficial since proper recovery would've helped my subsequent marathon results. Duly noted for the next time around!

Another point of Sarah's training had me simultaneously laughing and admiring her creativity. She found that the best way for her to get through some of the harder, cold and rainy runs was to pump up high-energy 80s music and use it as a soundtrack to …slay zombies. She created an entertaining sequence in her head where she was saving the day by fending off imaginary zombies (with a samurai sword, no less!) as she ran along her running path. Such a fun scenario could be the key to avoiding boredom on long runs.

Lastly, and most poignantly, Sarah found a way to make her marathon experience deeply meaningful. Having lived through tremendous family loss due to cancer in a very small window of time, she managed to add a note of positivity to the situation through her running effort. "I ran the marathon to raise money for Macmillan Cancer Research. Both my parents died of cancer within three months of each other, and so did my aunt, a year earlier. It was so motivating to see the donations come in. I ended up raising over 1,500 pounds [almost 2,000 US dollars], which felt great." Coming out of a devastating situation and finding a way for something good to shine through is truly exemplary.

In addition to the emotional factors, Sarah also had to deal with a sudden injury right at the end of her marathon training, because she twisted her ankle a week before the event. After resting for the days leading up to her race, she had a doctor wrap the ankle up and decided that if she ran carefully, she'd make it through. Towards the end of her 26point2, the emotions she was experiencing overcame the physical pain and propelled her to the finish. "I have to admit, the last mile of the race left me utterly defeated, and I felt like I couldn't go any further. I started thinking of my parents and aunt and how much people had donated, and whilst it wasn't the most dignified end to the marathon I imagined (I ended up crying that entire last mile), thinking of them got me to the end, so I'm grateful for that."

This grit and determination completely embody the marathon spirit. For more details about Sarah's marathon experience, please read on to see her questionnaire answers.

1. What time of day do you run and why?

"My training was quite erratic, really. I mainly trained

in the evenings, but my schedule was pretty much dictated by when the kids went to bed, and when my husband was around to look after them." Again, carving out the time to train with small children in the picture requires extensive logistical planning, but it absolutely can be done.

2. What do you typically eat before or after training sessions?

Sarah turned to "Marmite on toast before the run. It's the best! I can't live without the stuff. It is the one food source I would take with me on a desert island. It is salty and delicious. They say you either love it or you hate it. Clearly, I am a lover, and I genuinely feel bad for people who don't like it. They are missing out!"

Marmite is a distinctly British, yeast-based spread with a sharp savory tang that, as Sarah noted, tends to put people on vehemently opposing sides of the fence. There are two unmistakable camps, entailing either pure love for the product or a feeling of absolute disgust, and nobody waffles in the middle. As described by www.theguardian.com, "Marmite has a very distinctive flavor. The taste is so unique as to defy description, but think of a yeasty, salty, soy sauce-esque flavor with the consistency of old engine oil." That description alone makes it very clear as to why this product sparks controversy. A Marmite fan through and through, Sarah's preferred option is to spread it on toast, which she eats right before running to fulfill her craving.

3. What is your special, secret training tip?

Here's where the previously mentioned zombies come into play. "Whatever it is that makes your brain happy during cold and rainy runs, do it. Even if it means pretending you are a hero and running after zombies with really cheesy 80s music blaring through your earphones!" I love the idea of using creativity to reframe a challenging situation and make it enjoyable. Sarah is a highly creative person, and she found a distinctive way to let that mesh with her marathon training.

Additionally, Sarah turned to a resource that a friend gifted her time and time again throughout her training. "My best friend who has run tons of marathons bought me a book called *The Non-runner's Marathon Trainer* by David A. Whitsett, Forrest A. Dolgener and Tanjala Jo Kole. This book got me through the marathon! Whilst it is a little dated, and I had to do additional research on nutrition, it helped so much with the psychological and emotional issues that you will inevitably go through and better equipped me with how to deal with them."

Namely, Sarah found solace in the fact that the information in this book was not meant to be read all at once. "The book was beneficial to me because it was broken down into chapters in relation to the specific week of training, so I would read a chapter and then feel prepared for that coming week of running. It had motivational stories of other people who were at the same stage in training and tips on how they worked through the potential pitfalls." This is fitting because marathon training is about taking things one step at a time, not trying to do it all in one go.

4. Is there any cultural influence, or something going on in your personal life, that impacts your training?

Sarah overcame a last-minute injury to successfully complete her marathon. "There weren't really any major circumstances, but I did manage to twist my ankle a week before the marathon, as you do. It was a really nasty twist, and I thought I might not be able to run at all." A doctor wrapped her ankle the night before the race, and Sarah hoped for the best while trying to be mindful of her footing during the run. "I just had to be a lot more conscientious of it because I felt a lack of concentration might result in another twist during the race, which would have been *no bueno*."

5. Do you add any other exercise to your marathon preparation for cross training?

"No, I chose to do the bare minimum here."

6. How long is your marathon training cycle?

"I followed a 16-week training plan that involved running four times a week. Admittedly, I missed out on a fair few of the sessions…But I always made sure I did all the long runs! In hindsight, I may have enjoyed the actual race more had I done all the training…"

I can fully attest to Sarah's reasoning here. The only one of my marathons that I properly planned for by sticking to a training calendar turned out to be a Personal Best time and an absolute dream of a day. I barely felt my feet touch the ground until about the last ten minutes. The insight here is that **the time and effort put into the overall training is directly proportional to the level of enjoyment felt on race day**. Even if it's psychological, feeling prepared will lead to positive outcomes!

7. What do you eat for breakfast on the day of your marathon?

"I had a cup of tea and two slices of toast with peanut butter. I was staying at my friend's house, and they didn't have any Marmite, so peanut butter was the best substitute."

This breakfast worked in terms of providing the energy that Sarah needed; however, she craved the distinctive taste of her beloved Marmite! It's also ideal to keep the training and racing circumstances as similar as possible, so the option of bringing along a travel-sized version of the products consumed in training works well for destination races.

8. What did you eat and drink during the race? At what intervals?

Sarah opted for gels and water, consumed roughly about every half hour during the race, in addition to the aforementioned Jelly Babies candy which she says she munched on throughout the whole course. "I would slow down and walk the length of the water station sipping water and then start running again. I wasn't really too bothered about my finish time, I just wanted to actually finish." Combining the walking break with the hydration and refueling is a useful strategy. Less of your drink will be spilled, and you can dispose of the cup near the volunteers.

9. Deep thoughts: what was your mental preparation and focus throughout training and on race day? Do you use any outside running "distractions" (such as music, podcasts, running apps, etc.) while running?

The mental push Sarah got in her race was linked with her fundraising efforts for cancer research in her family's honor. Running can employ the legs, the brain, and also, as seen here, the heart.

10. What does your post-race period look like, both for recovery and celebrating? (Note: The celebration after crossing the finish line can serve as motivation that gets you through training and the race!)

The best-tasting beer of your entire life might just be consumed right after hitting the finish line of a marathon. "After I finished the race, I met up with my best friend and her wife who also ran the marathon, and we headed straight to a beer tent and drank a beer. It was hands down the absolute best beer I've ever had. A bunch of our friends came and joined us, and we had another beer and a burrito. Then we hobbled home, where I showered, got straight into my pajamas, and we ordered takeout curry."

Bonus Question: What should you NOT have done in your 26point2?

With dry humor, Sarah shares what to avoid. "Try not to twist your ankle before a big race. Or ever…"

The tenacity displayed throughout Sarah's racing experience is inspiring both on a physical and an emotional level. She ran with great intention and even somehow managed to incorporate zombie fun and burritos! The fans lining the marathon route played a part in getting Sarah through the race, as did her other fans that supported her fundraising and emotive marathon journey.

***

Sarah R., from the UK, has run in the UK and Austria

Mile 16: Train hard, run easy

Ben V.Z. from South Africa

Who knew that being passionate about saving the rhinoceros from extinction could lead to becoming a marathon runner? Ben V.Z. grew up near the famous Kruger National Park in South Africa and has dedicated his professional life to his love of wildlife through his work for a zoological society. He is now based out of a national park in Zambia and is in constant contact with awe-inspiring animals. It was here that he met athletic and animal-loving colleagues that were preparing to take on the 26point2 on the world stage of the London Marathon. Their goal was to raise awareness for the current and dire status of the rhino, which is dying out rapidly due to a variety of factors. The "Save the Rhinos" group strives to bring attention to their cause, garner support, and ultimately raise funds for rhino conservation.

After partaking in a prolonged marathon training cycle and traveling to London, Ben spontaneously made a big decision the night before his race. Ben's group connected with another team of marathoners from Zimbabwe who were also racing to benefit wildlife causes. "The Zimbabwe team had a guy running in a rhino suit. We were running to support rhinos, and I decided a night before the marathon that I needed to run in a suit as well." With that, Ben befriended a large theatrical rhino costume that weighed about 15 pounds (7 kilos). For better or worse, the two would run the entire marathon together to call even more attention to the cause of rhino conservation.

It was noticeably hot running a 26point2 inside the massive costume, and Ben had to adjust his form a bit as the suit bounced around as he ran which led him to trot very carefully.

Ben, however, was more than up to the challenge as his training had been even tougher. For his marathon prep, Ben shared that he "trained twice a day in the middle of the day when the sun was at its hottest and with a full sweat suit on in 100–105 degrees Fahrenheit [38–40 degrees Celsius]." He was, therefore, more than ready to take on the relatively cooler conditions in London and do the full race dressed as a burly rhino.

At the park in Zambia, Ben and his running buddies did their shorter workouts in more confined spaces because it was easier for the park rangers to control what was in their immediate area. They preferred to do their long runs outside of the park to lower the chances of crossing paths with the animals, for safety reasons. It may seem a bit surreal, but Ben has encountered warthogs, impalas, zebras, and even elephants on his runs. He recognizes it is best to stay far out of their way and to respect that he is, in fact, in their home. His training plan adapted to both his surroundings and to his belief in extremely challenging workouts.

1. What time of day do you run and why?

Ben strives to train midday and in the afternoon to be exposed to the hottest temperatures of the day. In some ways, this concept echoes what the elites do with high altitude training. When you push your body to the edge of its limits in a harsh environment, the idea is that on race day, if the conditions are less excruciating, then everything will seem effortless in comparison.

As noted earlier, all ideas presented in this book should be run by a doctor before incorporating them into a training plan, and this holds even more true with extreme training ideas that could potentially lead to more significant health complications.

2. What do you typically eat before or after training sessions?

Proving that even within the same region things can

vary immensely, Ben's diet is basically the polar opposite of what his fellow marathoner from South Africa, Alastair, eats (see Chapter 12). Ben eats meat about twice a day, and while he occasionally adds veggies to the mix, he tries to avoid eating carbohydrates in an effort to control his weight. For him, a simple formula to follow was to have a no-frills steak at mealtime, and he rarely deviated from that diet plan.

3. What is your special, secret training tip?

The whole basis of Ben's training ties in with his train hard, run easy philosophy. By making the training as demanding as possible, race day in comparison can be taken with a light approach. In his case, that approach allowed for a substantial addition in race gear in the form of the rhino suit, but since he had trained so hard, the race was still doable and even enjoyable.

4. Is there any cultural influence, or something going on in your personal life, that impacts your training?

Part of the drive for Ben's training was the companionship he found while running with colleagues and the shared love that they have for wildlife conservation. This shaped the whole marathon training experience, including race day, for Ben. "My training buddies were all running for the rhinos. They have been doing this a lot longer than me, and it is truly an inspiration to see how they work to keep these animals safe. My buddies are so fast and always run ahead of me, but in the end it's your own reason and your own journey that matters."

5. Do you add any other exercise to your marathon preparation for cross training?

Ben added standard squats and pushups to his training. Keeping in line with his philosophy, he did not shy away from tough strength-building sessions. "I was training really hard running and the days I didn't run, I did squats, to the extent of 400 in a single training session." Squats are a highly effective addition to a running program, especially in preparation for hill work.

6. How long is your marathon training cycle?

Ben describes the training cycle for his marathon as a much longer process than average — one full year — due to the fact that he had a parallel goal that went along with his training: he wanted to lose a significant amount of weight. With this goal in mind, he created a running and strength-training plan that worked in tandem with his colleagues' goal to run a marathon. He was able to shed the weight. He credits both running and improved eating habits to his admirable success.

7. What do you eat for breakfast on the day of your marathon?

A simple banana was Ben's pre-race fueling choice.

8. What did you eat and drink during the race? At what intervals?

Ben (and his rhino ;)) fueled and hydrated with water, Lucozade and gummy bears. I was unfamiliar with Lucozade and wanted to learn more about this beverage, so I went to the www.spectator.com.uk website, which informs that Lucozade was originally created in 1927 as a replenishing drink for people to recover from illness. It provides a boost of energy, as each serving has as much caffeine as a cup of tea and a sizeable amount of sugar, and many agree that its taste is simply unique. The website states that "The only thing Lucozade tastes of is Lucozade." Since the flavor of Lucozade seems to be beyond description, curious runners will have to try out this beverage for themselves and decide.

9. Deep thoughts: what was your mental preparation and focus throughout training and on race day? Do you use any outside running "distractions" (such as music, podcasts, running apps, etc.) while running?

While Ben listened to lots of music during his training runs, during his 26point2 he found it more rewarding to get rid of his headphones. "People were motivating me like crazy," he said, and he wanted to soak it all in.

10. What does your post-race period look like, both for recovery and celebrating? (Note: The celebration after crossing the finish line can serve as motivation that gets you through training and the race!)

There was little relaxation following Ben's marathon efforts; immediately after finishing his race, he was already thinking ahead to the next opportunity he would have to be able to do it again! He feels deeply connected to what he and his teammates accomplished, both personally and for the rhinos. He is determined that he will go at it again, for the same cause and train even harder for better results the next time around.

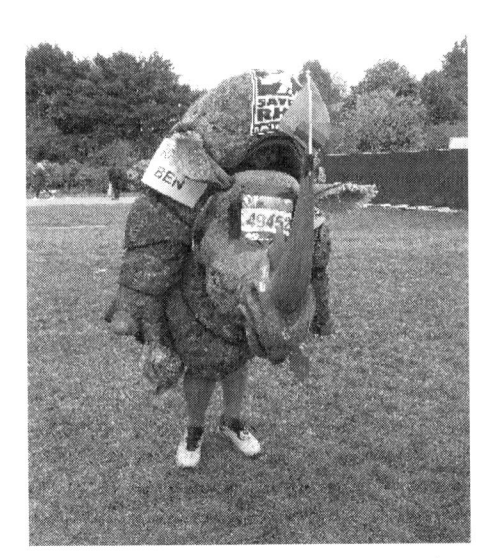

"Rhino Ben" and his medal post-marathon. Photo courtesy of Doug Goodman and Save the Rhino International

The London Marathon is an iconic and inspiring event, and the opportunity to run in that environment greatly impacted Ben. According to him, it was simply, "Fantastic! Everyone is motivating you and was very friendly. It's a great day out." Runner's World magazine deems the London Marathon the most popular run of all times, with over 414,000 marathoners vying to get in yearly. Tightly linked to charity endeavors, it raises millions each year for a wide variety of beneficial initiatives and unites the entire city, and even the world, through its international runners that exude positive energy and sportsmanship. Many happily do so for charitable causes.

Ben's cause, specifically, is a critical one. It's been said that there are more runners participating in the London Marathon than rhinos left in the world, and the situation is getting more precarious with each passing year. The rhino-clad runners in the London Marathon serve as an unmissable message which is found in large block print on the runners' costumes: "Save The Rhino!"

While the marathon was admittedly a challenge for Ben, due in part to the added effort he faced while running with the rhino suit on, he triumphed and only has positive things to say about the experience. To prepare for the next 26point2, he now wears a 22-pound (10-kilo) backpack on all of his long runs. Running the full marathon in the rhino suit, in comparison, should feel like a breeze, and doing so again in the electrifying atmosphere of the London Marathon, for the benefit of rhinos everywhere, is a true inspiration.

***

Benjamin V.Z., from South Africa, has run in the UK and Zambia

Mile 17: Putting the Fly in Your Stride

Kristin S. from USA

Boutique fitness studios have become increasingly popular in the United States in recent years. These specialized fitness centers offer classes that range from barre workouts to Pilates to spinning. Living in Europe, I am not so familiar with this newer trend, so I decided to dig a bit deeper. According to www.mindbody.io, such studios are known for "offering workouts or services with a high experiential factor, smaller, more intimate class sizes, and strong brand association. Not to mention a sense of camaraderie that can't be ignored. The notion 'vibe attracts your tribe' is applicable here."

A tribe of runners based out of Minneapolis, USA, now has the opportunity to prepare for marathons in an innovative and new way. The vibe at a new running studio is inclusive and inspirational while remaining highly results-oriented. All this is thanks to an initiative carried out by multi-hyphenate American marathoner-entrepreneur-mom, Kristin S.

In 2016, Kristin noticed that the boutique fitness studio sector offered a wide array of workouts, but realized a void existed and saw an opportunity to bring her beloved sport of running into the fold. This is how Fly Feet Running came to be. This group fitness studio aims to "Inspire people to chase the best version of themselves."

Both Kristin and Fly Feet subscribe to a holistic approach. The main focuses are the mechanics of running, strength building through interval training, optimal diet strategies, efficient stretching techniques, and recovery. Fly Feet Running plays a key role in Kristin's marathon success as of late. Due to this system, she has been able to qualify for and run in the Boston Marathon for the first time in 15 years.

Numerous distance runners in the Fly Feet tribe also report that after adding two to three Fly Feet classes to their regular weekly routine, they get remarkable changes in their finishing times and even achieve elusive PRs. Kristin feels that this is because Fly Feet brings the science behind the sport to the masses in a personalized way. There are at least two coaches on hand during every Fly Feet class to keep a close eye on each runner's mechanics and form so they can obtain the best results.

What can someone training for a marathon expect at a Fly Feet workout session? "Our classes are 60 minutes long and "HIIT"-based (High-Intensity Interval Training). The class is split between running and strength training. We use all functional movements so that you not only become a better athlete, but as a human you move well and stay injury free. Runners are notorious for hamstring injuries due to weakness in both the hamstrings and gluts. Building strength allows you to build power and speed, and most importantly, stave off injuries.

Every day the workout is different, but each day you'll do some short running intervals on the treadmill [treadmill work is helpful for running coaches to closely examine any issues with gait] and strength work on the floor — think pushups, pull ups, burpees, kettlebell swings, chest press, and squats, all for functional movement. We do all the things that make you a better runner — sprints, hills, repeats, strength training, etc., — but that runners don't like to do on their own," shares Kristin.

The classes improve negative issues that many runners try to resolve. Lack of strength or mobility can result in problems such as improper heel striking. At Fly Feet, there is a constructive focus on correcting issues related to form by breaking down simple motions. "It's much easier to diagnose faults in running mechanics in scaled-down movement. We focus on mechanics by analyzing basic movements first, assessing faults, and determining fixes. If we can get people to **move well in a scaled down version of running, for example, lunging, squatting, or walking, then it will translate to much better running mechanics**."

So, how can you benefit from this running tribe if you are training for a marathon and don't have access to this studio? Incorporate a few key Fly Feet strategies seen below, and then do as I'm doing, which is to plan for a future visit to Minneapolis in order to learn from these innovative running professionals in person.

Tips gleaned from Fly Feet:

- Chalk up your goals. Each participant at a Fly Feet session writes that day's goal on the ground in chalk. This simple act keeps the goal present and binds you closer to it. I've taken to chalking up, for example, ten hill series at the bottom of a steep hill (I'll just mark a small "10" on the ground, as I'm the only one that needs to know what it stands for). Then I splash away that goal with a bit of water when finished. It feels great to commit to something and later be able to wipe out that accomplishment when it's reached.

- Engage a tribe! Find a group that also sees the advantage of adding strength training to a workout and get in the habit of incorporating things like squats or burpees that can be done with no equipment after (or during!) a run.

- Analyze your gait. Coaches, podiatrists, yoga instructors or even experienced employees at running stores that have studied body mechanics can pick up on flaws when you run or stride, so ask around your community where you can locate an informed person and try to get some feedback. At some forward-thinking shops that sell running shoes, they even hook up cameras to a treadmill as you try shoes out, so your stride can be observed in slow motion. Alternatively, a friend could make a video of you in action.

- Check out www.flyfeetrunning.com, Fly Feet's highly informative website, for videos about strengthening, training, stretching, and motivation, as well as links to diet ideas and recipes for runners.

It's no surprise that Fly Feet Running adds a vital element to Kristin's marathon experience but read on to find out the other components that she relies on.

1. What time of day do you run and why?

"Typically, I run first thing in the morning. It's my favorite time of the day. I feel best in the morning."

2. What do you typically eat before or after training sessions?

Kristin doesn't vary her training diet from her regular habits too much since her approach to nutrition is well thought out for health and performance. Her norm is to eat whole foods and avoid anything highly processed. "I don't eat bars or energy drinks, or anything processed before/during/after running as I find that they upset my stomach. After a run, I love a huge cup of coffee and grapes!"

3. What is your special, secret training tip?

"Put in the work if you want to have a good race." Simple and to the point, this message is actually no secret. In fact, it's been heavily acknowledged in this very book because running long distances successfully always circles back to putting in the work. Kristin also advocates self-care to recover from her high mileage in the form of weekly massages.

4. Is there any cultural influence, or something going on in your personal life, that impacts your training?

"Running has always been a release for me. It allows me to clear my head, work through problems, and feel good about myself, and life in general. **I have always used running as a mental health tool** and enjoy long runs, so marathon training just gives me more of what I love."

She also notes that she had to take special care while keeping up her running in some areas of the world due to the cultural context. For example, when she was a volunteer for two years in El Salvador, Central America, she was living on a coffee plantation. Since physical labor was the basis of many people's jobs in the area, the concept of going for a run and exerting more energy seemed foreign to many locals.

Kristin felt it was even stranger for her to be running as a woman. According to her, at that time in her village, many women didn't usually even go outside alone, much less run. She developed a thick skin against any comments and stares and carried on.

5. Do you add any other exercise to your marathon preparation for cross training?

"I was able to get exceptionally faster much later in my running career (at 40, after three kids) after integrating high-intensity interval training to my routine. Classes at Fly Feet push you to do things that you'd never do on your own such as sprint repeats, hills, and strength work to stave off injury. I got faster and stayed injury-free by integrating two to three speed and strength workouts a week. I also qualified for Boston for a second time, 15 years later!"

6. How long is your marathon training cycle?

Kristin dedicates 18 weeks to marathon preparation, which allows her to steadily ramp up her mileage and incorporate the longer runs gradually. She believes in doing interval training year-round to stay strong and ward off injury.

7. What do you eat for breakfast on the day of your marathon?

"If I'm home, two eggs and one avocado plus coffee because that is what I always eat. If I'm traveling to a race, I'll do a banana plus one piece of peanut butter toast because that's what I eat on the road." Having thought out a meal plan for both home and on the road is smart. It takes the guesswork out of what a hotel breakfast might offer and leaves you one less decision to make the morning of race day.

8. What did you eat and drink during the race? At what intervals?

"I only drink water during the race. I never skip a water stop, even if it's just a sip. I carry an Rx bar with me but almost never eat it. It's just for insurance. As I mentioned previously, the processed stuff usually hurts my stomach, but I find that Rx bars are better. I like that they are simple ingredients — a fairly clean ingredient deck." (www.rxbar.com)

9. Deep thoughts: what was your mental preparation and focus throughout training and on race day? Do you use any outside running "distractions" (such as music, podcasts, running apps, etc.) while running?

Kristin's focus while running is only possible for runners with great control and insight into their personal limits. "I do a 10-mile threshold run every week where I push myself to the edge. During a race, I try and stay just below that threshold. This takes a lot of mental training. **Your body does what your mind tells it to do.**"

Additionally, Kristin runs with music (hip hop!) or a podcast. Most frequently, she looks to podcasts that are insightful for entrepreneurs such as "How I Built This" or "Masters of Scale." I would not be surprised to hear Kristin herself, with her insights regarding running and creation of Fly Feet, featured on one of these very podcasts in the near future.

10. What does your post-race period look like, both for recovery and celebrating? (Note: The celebration after crossing the finish line can serve as motivation that gets you through training and the race!)

The Fly Feet philosophy attaches great importance to

personalized, meaningful recovery, and more so after a big endeavor such as a marathon. In the big picture, allowing for restoration is a commitment to wellbeing. Some ways to achieve this are to listen to your body and allow it adequate time to heal. Specifically, Fly Feet recommends aiming for a few chosen days of light movement at about 50–60 percent capacity after a 26point2.

Bonus Question: What should you NOT have done in your 26point2?

"My first marathon (many, many years ago) I wore cotton socks. That was a bad idea." Kristin is not a fan of cotton socks because she thinks they were responsible for the numerous blisters she ended up with at that race. She suggests that runners try out socks made of a synthetic blend. Her favorite socks come from a brand called Thorlo (www.thorlo.com) because they provide cushioning and don't cause chafing.

Kristin highlights her insights on marathon running and life with the following: "There is power in being vulnerable and tackling something that you're not sure you can do. If we can get people to take on their fears in the studio, we believe that it translates to their lives. We believe that fear of failure holds us back. Failure gives us something to reach for and work for and conquer. We believe that from that struggle comes courage and confidence and willingness to keep pushing. We believe we can do it."

***

"One can choose to go back to safety or toward growth. Growth must be chosen, again and again, fear must be overcome again and again."

–Abraham Maslow

***

The idea that running magic deriving from hard work

later translates into real-life success is an inspirational concept worth chasing down.

***

**Kristin S., from USA, has run in USA
(15 marathons including Boston, Chicago, and New York),
El Salvador, Uganda, and all over Asia and Europe**

Mile 18: With Swiss Precision

Ina V. from Romania

Ina V. is a multifaceted Romanian runner with extensive experience in marathons, trail runs, and triathlons. She currently lives in Switzerland, so many of her training sessions are done surrounded by stunning mountainous scenery (I know this first-hand as she and her partner Klaus send awe-inspiring pictorial updates of their running adventures to a group chat of runners that I belong to). Ina is also a committed professional with a demanding job, but she has found a way to incorporate her dedication to the office with her passion for running. She does so with the detailed precision that her adopted country is famous for.

I know what you are thinking…demanding professional life, successful and precise runner…so how does this work? Take a look at a sample of her workweek. "I take advantage of my lunch break to run: one day trail, one day forest run with hills, one day intervals, and one day 30 minutes with no break." Ina feels that even a quick run of 30–40 minutes helps her to push a reset button in her day and face the afternoon with renewed energy.

These workouts are topped off with evening runs in the company of a training group she belongs to that offers controlled pace runs, and she always saves the weekend for well-planned training sessions or racing adventures with Klaus. During the winter weekends, the time allotted for outdoor running is shortened due to lack of light, but they still get in extensive workouts in nature both on Saturday and Sunday. In summer, they alternate between longer biking adventures and exploring beautiful Alpine running routes. Ina is known to jump into freezing mountain lakes to cap off the runs with swims as well. Both Ina and Klaus are avid travelers, and often incorporate running tourism into both their business and personal travel plans.

Everything Ina and Klaus do involving sports seems highly organized, meticulously planned and well thought out. Ina also gauges the effort expended in her carefully-planned runs. She employs her Garmin heart rate monitor through her phone and listens for indications of her heart rate to adjust to her targets accordingly. She notes that these values alter when she runs mountain trails (where she'll generally have a lower target heart rate) and when on the road where she pushes her speed.

Ina has also learned exactly how her body burns fuel. She's studied the most effective calorie targets, as well as the quantities and types of protein and carbohydrates that best serve her while participating in physical activities. Ina knows the amount of carbs that her body typically has "on reserve" and feels her performance is better while working within that range. This information is helpful for anticipating drops in energy.

While running all over the world, Ina has shared in some race day experiences that seem both charming and culturally relevant:

- In France, they handed out delicate Madeleine butter cakes for a mid-race treat;
- In Milan, members of the military served tea to the runners upon finishing;
- In Lucerne, Switzerland, she recalled with delight costumed bands for Carnival performing along the racecourse;
- In Jungfrau, Switzerland (a celebrated mountain race that starts in Interlaken), she noted the picturesque tall Alp horns played against the stunning mountain backdrop. According to the

- Lonely Planet, this race is "A beautiful brute... Breathtaking in every sense," and Rivella, a traditional milk-whey soft drink thought to help with recovery, is served;
- She remembers Zurich, Switzerland as a very fast, practical and well-laid-out marathon that was remarkably orderly and quiet, which Ina said, "allows you to focus;"
- In mountain marathons around Switzerland, the race times feel no longer relevant as runners stop at rest stations for cheese, cured meat, and conversation. People take the time for a leisurely chat and enjoy the moment in nature with the company of fellow runners and local hosts;
- Barcelona, Spain, evokes a feeling of participation in an Olympic-style marathon as the entire city pours out for enthusiastic fan support worthy of the international games;
- In Boston, USA, Ina did not let the grueling weather conditions of the 2018 marathon — thought by some to be the worst in the event's history due to the rain, wind and cold — negatively impact her. She sloshed through with heavy soaked shoes and felt a special appreciation for the crowds cheering her on despite the horrible conditions.

Read on for more details about how Ina approaches her running.

1. What time of day do you run and why?

During the workweek, Ina aims for four lunchtime runs with two added evening workouts. She goes for very high mileage over the weekends and often does all-day running adventures. How long she'll go will vary if she is preparing for a big race or not. Her weekend runs hover around six hours or more.

2. What do you typically eat before or after training sessions?

Ina doesn't change her diet too much in relation to her running program. "We just go running and eat normal food," she states with practicality. She creates space in her diet for treats and especially enjoys local baked goods called *Bibers*, which are a kind of cookie stuffed with marzipan. When she has a particularly long or hard run, she'll employ what she refers to as "plastic food," which is basically processed food that comes in wrappers. This kind of food is not her first preference, but it is portable and convenient to eat on the move.

3. What is your special, secret training tip?

Ina keeps her advice pragmatic here: "Just go for the best you can."

4. Is there any cultural influence, or something going on in your personal life, that impacts your training?

When Ina first left her home country Romania, she discovered it was not easy to get the medication she used for the treatment of a liver condition she had in her new city. In Romania, this treatment was available without a prescription, but in her new residence, it needed a doctor's authorization. Her new doctor told her to take up sports instead of relying on the pills and that's how she started running, which she says has now evolved into what she calls the "holy hour" of her day.

5. Do you add any other exercise to your marathon preparation for cross training?

"We go swimming, biking or cross-country skiing." The natural beauty of Switzerland serves as an envy-inducing backdrop for all of these activities, and the mountains allow for an extended season of snow sports.

6. How long is your marathon training cycle?

As her fitness baseline is typically so high, Ina requires no specialized marathon training. The only change she'll make before a marathon is to set apart time for a little rest. "I try to have a two-day running break beforehand." Ina also recognizes that her motivation for participation in this distance varies. Since she often opts for longer races, she might participate in the 26point2 simply to join friends that are also running or to see the streets of a new city from the perspective of the racecourse.

7. What do you eat for breakfast on the day of your marathon?

"I have learned that I have to be careful. I drink coffee, no milk, no sugar, and eat some sweets, but nothing with honey." Ina has determined that for her, eating fruit directly before a run leads to an upset stomach, so she tries to avoid it the day before and morning of the race. Additionally, milk, when combined with energy products that she uses later in the run, leads to the same issue, so she makes sure not to have any before a race.

8. What did you eat and drink during the race? At what intervals?

Here, Ina comments on her beverage selection: "Water always, and isotonic drinks. I like Red Bull if they have it and when finishing the event, I enjoy a cola."

9. Deep thoughts: what was your mental preparation and focus throughout training and on race day? Do you use any outside running "distractions" (such as music, podcasts, running apps, etc.) while running?

Ina focuses on her heart rate monitoring system through her phone to keep her target pace but uses no other apps or music.

10. What does your post-race period look like, both for recovery and celebrating? (Note: The celebration after crossing the finish line can serve as motivation that gets you through training and the race!)

"As I do not have much breakfast beforehand, I love the

finish line food and I am totally unhappy when there is little or nothing to eat, or if I am sick and cannot eat. I do not take too much because I think of the people running behind me, but I am happy that I finally get something to eat."

Bonus Question: What should you NOT have done in your 26point2?

Ina feels that runners should not underestimate the importance of a visit to the bathroom before a race and the line you might encounter there (which translates to time lost for warm ups and stretching). It should also be noted that a mid-race bathroom break probably won't unfavorably impact your results. As Ina points out, even the winner of the Boston Marathon in 2018 waited as her running mate stopped for a quick bathroom break. Desi Linden cemented herself in history as a hero running partner for waiting while her teammate popped into the loo. The takeaway is **don't stress out too much about bathroom breaks in general; stop if needed so as to run comfortably**.

Ina's running events around the world and in the beautiful Swiss mountains at home involve precise planning. She is also very meticulous when describing her involvement with running and wishes to make it clear that, "I do not like the words training, athlete, and competition. I would replace them with activity, participant, and event." Her belief is that the athlete label should be reserved for someone with elite status that has made major sacrifices over the course of a lifetime for his or her sport. She therefore considers herself an economist that carries out running activities and participates in events.

As seen by her regular visits to the podium at highly competitive races, Ina is clearly a very successful participant! As with most aspects of her running, she just prefers to be precise with the terminology that she uses to describe her endeavors. In this connection, precision has proven to form a part of outstanding running.

***
Ina V., from Romania, has run in Romania, Austria, Croatia, France, Greece, Italy, Spain, Switzerland, and USA

Mile 19: If You Build It, They Will Come

Iván F.R. from Spain

Iván F.R. shares the marathon experiences he has gleaned through years of running in Sevilla, Spain, and throughout the region of Andalusia. When he became the founder and coach of a training club called "Heroes Without Capes," he discovered that this role provided him incredible motivation and an ideal way to meet his personal running goals. He organizes biweekly runs for his group and focuses on data-based speed series programs. The shared experience of group training spurs him on, and the results are incredibly positive. A healthy dose of swimming and strength work for cross training is added to his routine to prevent injury. Biking is also a fundamental part of his athletic endeavors because Iván enjoys participating in triathlons.

The Heroes Without Capes team provides a far-reaching social component for its members, but its main purpose is to act as a driver to achieve optimal training. With a laugh, Iván shares, "I had to start my own club in order to really train!" and he goes on to clarify that when his fellow team members are counting on him to lead his demanding late evening workouts, he will never skip them and gives his all at every single session.

The dedication with which Iván approaches his training commitments says a lot about him as a person. His marathon training cycles are well-studied and highly organized. They are demanding yet fun, as he realizes the importance of having a good time with his group. As a leader, he is supportive, highly engaged, and generous with sharing his knowledge. The following answers illustrate Iván's belief that "The marathon is life itself." It goes without saying that how he lives is how he runs.

1. What time of day do you run and why?

Iván and his fellow heroes start their training after work around 7:30 or 8:00 p.m., but some runners tend to show up later. In southern Spain a typical workday can finish as late as 9:00 p.m. or even 10:00 p.m. A midday break for lunch and siesta from 2:00 to 5:00 p.m. is the norm in some workplaces, so the finishing times are rarely early. Getting a run in after work can often be on the later side. Saturday morning runs also form a part of his regular training week.

2. What do you typically eat before or after training sessions?

Before Iván's weeknight training sessions, he has a snack after he finishes work. He usually opts to eat something light, such as fruit or half a sandwich, but he makes sure to have a balanced dinner after he runs. "At dinner, after working out, I try to combine protein with carbohydrates and always have large portions of vegetables as well."

3. What is your special, secret training tip?

Here Iván has an insightful strategy that involves his sharp attention to data. While preparing for a marathon, he creates new formulas for his different workouts. Specifically, he studies what his target heart rate should be for optimal results and aims to be very precise about hitting it. He applies this knowledge to both speed workouts and longer runs and has made a standout discovery. By targeting certain heart rates, he has more effective training sessions. His total volume of training has reduced, but his performance level has notably increased. He is happy to say that he and his team are now "reaching higher goals and better times with less effort," since he's found a way that works for him to train smarter.

"For many years, I'd run a lot of kilometers without controlling my pace. My focus was just to run longer and longer. Fortunately, I changed my training strategy about three years ago. I focus on my heart rate and am now able to achieve my goals."

4. Is there any cultural influence, or something going on in your personal life, that impacts your training?

A little love goes a long way. Iván has a partner that shares his love of running and can match both his strides and his passion for training. He claims this is a great advantage that helps to pave the way for successful results. "The fact that my girlfriend is in our training club has a really positive influence on me; she's a great part of the group, and it's so important to me to have her full support. She really understands why I spend so much of my free time training." In fact, she's often right there with him in her free time as she works out with the group as much as possible. This concept ties in with a quote from an anonymous source: "Love, like fire, cannot subsist without continual movement."

***

"Love, like fire, cannot subsist without continual movement."

–Anonymous

***

5. Do you add any other exercise to your marathon preparation for cross training?

Since Iván also participates in triathlons, he logically turns to swimming and biking to round out his running workouts. He also believes in the importance of strength training and incorporates a lot of varied strength work to his training plan by using weightlifting circuits at the gym.

6. How long is your marathon training cycle?

The structure of Iván's tried and true training cycle does not typically change, although the content of his workouts may vary. He might try out new strategies to strive for improved results. For a marathon training cycle, he progressively adds distance to his long runs over the course of two months. He pays close attention to his effort level and aims to run at 75–80 percent of his maximum heart rate capacity. He also adds in some speed workouts, and during these he aims for 85–90 percent when doing both 1,000- and 2,000-meter intervals.

7. What do you eat for breakfast on the day of your marathon?

Iván underscores the importance of eating exactly the same thing on race day that he eats throughout his training. No deviations should be allowed. "If you try to eat something really different than your normal diet and what your body is generally used to, you might feel really awful. This can derail the months of hard work and effort leading up to the race," he says. Breakfast for him consists of a cup of coffee and toasted bread with turkey slices, tomato and *queso fresco* which is a mild white cheese. He aims to eat 45 minutes to an hour before running.

8. What did you eat and drink during the race? At what intervals?

"I drink water and energy drinks every 5 to 10 km. How often I drink depends on how hot it is and how thirsty I am. I also make sure to have four glucose gels on me during the marathon. Two of them are fast-acting with added caffeine, and two are caffeine-free. I always make sure to save one of the caffeinated ones for the last few kilometers of the race in case I need that extra boost."

9. Deep thoughts: what was your mental preparation and focus throughout training and on race day? Do you use any outside running "distractions" (such as music, podcasts, running apps, etc.) while running?

"All the mental preparation for the marathon takes place in the long runs leading up to it. I sometimes listen to music, really inspiring music, but the best company is a running buddy that holds the same pace. I also always rely on a GPS with a heart rate monitor to be aware of my level of exertion."

10. What does your post-race period look like, both for recovery and celebrating? (Note: The celebration after crossing the finish line can serve as motivation that gets you through training and the race!)

"After the race, I just want to be with my family and friends and do whatever I feel like…more so if the race went well!!!"

Bonus Question: What should you NOT have done in your 26point2?

Iván was so excited about his first marathon that he wanted to wear all of the gear he got in the race goodie bag, including the brand-new T-shirt and shorts. He was only 23 years old and credits enthusiasm (and naïveté) to this plan, which did not pan out well in the end.

He ended up with angry red chafing from the new and unfamiliar running fabric. We've all heard the sensible advice to avoid wearing new clothing, but it's easy to be tempted to try something new at the last minute. A savvy move is to **plan out what you'll wear a week in advance and set your trusted outfit aside for the morning of your competition**. This way, there is one less decision to make the morning of the race. For Iván, this was a painful case of "live and learn," and he is happy to pass along the lesson so that others can avoid such an unpleasant situation.

There's no doubt that Iván's Heroes Without Capes team members have heard this specific tip and benefitted from it, and all the other shared knowledge from their leader. Iván built the group to help others in their running pursuits, and in the end his personal running goals greatly benefitted as well.

***
Iván F.R., from Spain, has run in Spain

Mile 20: Running towards the sun
Jean-Marie W. from Luxembourg

Jean-Marie W. hails from the tiny nation of Luxembourg, but much of his marathon running has taken place on an international stage. From dodging donkeys on racecourses in Morocco to being tightly corralled into starting corridors in Italy, for Jean-Marie, diversity is a key part of the experience. If possible, he likes to organize large and lively groups of up to 20–30 running friends to partake in the races. This makes for great post-race celebrations where sharing stories often results in a raucous clamor.

Another strategy that Jean-Marie employs involves making the most of the climatic conditions that he trains in. Although Jean-Marie no longer lives in his native Luxembourg, he is still based out of a northern European city which features long, dark and dreary winters.. These can be challenging and quickly deflate motivation, but Jean-Marie has a philosophy that embraces positive thinking, and literally "running into the light."

Jean-Marie shares that on early morning runs he loves to chase the first light of day. "In winter, I can see the daylight opening up before me as I run. Psychologically, that is so much better than running into the darkness." Even on the coldest and darkest days of winter, the black and inky night lightens up a bit in the morning. Those streaks of color, however faint, can be uplifting when they break through the dark sky, first cautiously and then with greater force. In those the first glimmers of light, Jean-Marie finds the inspiration to move forward with his run and with the new day. He strongly believes that witnessing those moments makes it worth getting out of bed on a cold, bleak morning.

Throughout the research phase of this book, I tried out many of the gems of advice that the seasoned runners featured on these pages highlighted. I can confirm that Jean-Marie's philosophy holds true, especially when the temperatures, and motivation levels, are running low. It might be found in the faint outline of a cloud, or a blur of green in the distance, but those first glowing traces of light seen when out on a frigid run are indubitably uplifting. The ultimate prize awarded to committed morning runners is a display of stunning colors in the sunrise that follows.

Like trip souvenirs from travels, Jean-Marie has collected a variety of interesting tactics to help him stay on track with his running. When I asked him to share a few, this is what he told me:

1. What time of day do you run and why?

Jean-Marie exclusively trains very early in the morning. This is in part due to the long and unpredictable hours of his working life, which often eliminate the possibility of any kind of evening workout. The takeaway here is to **run when you know you can**. Being able to carve out that time is the first consideration, and other factors like the weather come next.

2. What do you typically eat before or after training sessions?

Due to the pre-dawn wake-up time, Jean-Marie doesn't eat right away and, time permitting, he savors his breakfast after the run. If he's in a rush to get to the office, he may skip breakfast altogether, but if he has a bit more time, he'll eat some bread with jam.

It's interesting to note that when Jean-Marie is in a more

serious and results-focused training mode, he alters his diet to include homemade smoothies with a variety of healthy ingredients that aid recovery after his runs. He noted that there was a peak in this more focused running period about five years ago, and now his running routine is more relaxed. Diet is an important factor to adjust while considering performance goals.

3. What is your special, secret training tip?

"I run with friends most of the time. This helps motivate me during harder moments." Jean-Marie attributes so much importance to running with others that he even maintains that, "It's better to have a slow run with a friend than a fast run alone." He organizes group runs that accommodate his early schedule and usually has no problem enticing runners to join him, even at 6:30 a.m. in the morning.

Jean-Marie also recognizes the importance of a full recovery after pushing himself on long runs. "Recuperation, and especially getting enough sleep after a long run, is the most important part of training for me."

4. Is there any cultural influence, or something going on in your personal life, that impacts your training?

"Running was my way to integrate into new cultures. I now know so many people from very different parts of society because of running. Training isn't affected by life circumstances, but quite the opposite, my life is affected (in a positive way) by my training. It was a constant and a way to make friends."

5. Do you add any other exercise to your marathon preparation for cross training?

A common occurrence for many runners is to recognize the importance of stretching within a training cycle, but not actually stretch after a workout. "I do some stretching, but not enough. I have to do this more often—I'll try it again next year." Stretching can be equated to the flossing of fitness. Everyone knows it should be done, but for some reason it always seems like a challenge to actually do it. Start small and get in the habit of adding a stretching session of even five minutes, which is both beneficial and restorative.

6. How long is your marathon training cycle?

Marathon runners who race frequently can potentially be in constant and consecutive training mode. Jean-Marie says, "After a marathon is before a marathon. I run three to four marathons a year, so the last marathon was the first long run for the training of the next marathon."

7. What do you eat for breakfast on the day of your marathon?

Here Jean-Marie points out a perspective that is often overlooked. The focus of what one eats on race day, or at a pasta party held the night before, always garners a lot of attention. Yet Jean-Marie feels he gets his actual fuel on race day from what he has stored up over the three to four days leading up to the marathon. On race day, he will eat his standard small breakfast, which consists of two mini bread rolls with honey or jam eaten at least three hours before the race start. He makes a valid point that "Race day itself is too late to fix something with nutrition."

Shifting the focus from the 24 hours right before a race to several days before the marathon is an idea that is worth keeping in mind. The same thinking can be applied to other aspects of race day and could in fact alleviate some stress. For example, if you are worried you will not sleep very well the night before your race, you can proactively try to provide rest for your body over the course of the three or four nights leading up to your marathon by going to bed early and getting in some naps and extra rest during the day. This way, you are not trying to compensate for any sleep deficits the night before and hopefully will find you feel well-rested when you wake up on race day regardless of the actual sleep you got.

It's also important not to stress out too much in the

event of poor sleep quality the night before the 26point2. Due to abundant nervous energy, many runners are in the same boat and find themselves restless and unable to fall into a deep sleep right before race day. One elite runner manages to find solace in this widespread situation. She is an insomniac and the one night that she makes peace with her nocturnal tossing and turning is the night before a 26point2, since she figures that all her fellow marathoners are feeling the same way. **By making sure that the week leading up to the marathon has overall good sleep quality, the fear of not resting well the night before can be abated**.

8. What did you eat and drink during the race? At what intervals?

After the midway point of his marathon, Jean-Marie will eat some gels or an energy bar (typically a PowerBar). He looks for isotonic beverages at the aid stops because he feels he loses a lot of salts due to high perspiration and seeks to restore that loss. The actual quantity he consumes varies due to how hot it is during the race.

9. Deep thoughts: what was your mental preparation and focus throughout training and on race day? Do you use any outside running "distractions" (such as music, podcasts, running apps, etc.) while running?

During training, Jean-Marie sometimes tries to listen to music, but that usually doesn't last very long. "Normally, within a very short time, I run into somebody I can run and talk with."

10. What does your post-race period look like, both for recovery and celebrating? (Note: The celebration after crossing the finish line can serve as motivation that gets you through training and the race!)

"After a race, I normally celebrate with friends who just ran as well. We call it ARP (After Race Party). We do that party every time after a marathon. Normally the group reaches up to

20–30 people. We tell each other all the great stories from during the race."

In certain parts of the world, Jean-Marie and his running friends have a lot to recount! They have noticed fun and highly varied elements of the marathon experience on race days, based on the different cultures in which they are running. According to Jean-Marie, in Spain you'll find very packed streets and tight narrow race lanes. "It makes you feel like you're participating in the Tour de France!" In Slovakia, an original and energetic powerhouse sweet was offered at kilometer 30 (mile 18.5) in the form of a delicious chocolate-covered banana. In the USA, innovative sticks with Vaseline on the tip (to reduce chafing) were handed out to racers. And in Morocco, Jean-Marie and his pack of running friends recalled with amazement how they had to race through 2–3 km (1.5 miles) of loud and hectic traffic on the racecourse which featured motorcycles that surged among the runners and loaded cargo donkeys that they needed to maneuver around. The successful navigation of that particular 26point2 was definitely cause for celebration!

Bonus Question: What should you NOT have done in your 26point2?

Jean-Marie recommends not to start out too hard or too fast with a marathon training cycle to avoid burnout throughout the process.

The takeaway from Jean-Marie's enlivened conversation about his international marathon experiences is that when done among running friends, even avoiding race day surprises such as dodging uninvited donkeys on the course will result in a good time. Friends make every experience better, but if you have to go out alone, you can always strive to be inspired by the first hints of the sun on a dark morning.

***

Jean-Marie W., from Luxembourg, has run in

**Luxembourg, Austria,
Cyprus, France, Germany, Italy, Morocco, Norway,
Slovakia, Spain, Switzerland, the UK, and USA**

Mile 21: 26point2 Equals Three Half Marathons

Željko Š. from Croatia

Željko Š., or Z as I have called him over the years, and his huge high-energy pup Luna were among my first running buddies when I moved to Vienna, Austria. When I think back to the welcoming runs he organized for newcomers, I remember that at one he even slowed down to a snail's pace on his bike to lead me to the best route home from our group's meeting spot as I jogged alongside. Z provided a warm reception to the Vienna running scene while also giving a preview of the friendly and welcoming ethos found in his home country, Croatia.

I've visited Croatia on numerous occasions because I'm drawn to its beautiful beaches and I'm convinced that there's no color in the world quite like the impossibly deep blue of the Adriatic Sea. The seafood and warm, fun-loving people that live there also add to the experience. Even on short visits, welcoming locals will start to recognize you as you stroll (or run) about and are happy to throw out a *Dobro jutro*! good morning greeting.

I even had the great pleasure of crossing the finish line of an exciting race in a Roman amphitheater that is still intact in Pula, Croatia. The experience of completing the race in the stunning Arena, which is an imposing arched structure that sat up to 26,000 spectators, is unparalleled. It was easy to imagine a chariot racing alongside me as I sped to the finish line.

Z has had his share of singular racing experiences in countries all over central Europe. Read on to get a picture of the details and how he prepares for them.

1. What time of day do you run and why?

Z, like many other professionals, turns to the after-work hours to get a run in. The time of day he does his training sessions is not as noteworthy as how much thought he puts into them. I can confirm this because he has extensively learned a network of intricate running paths that crisscross a vast wooded area. To the benefit of Z's running groups, he is happy to share everything he knows about these routes.

2. What do you typically eat before or after training sessions?

In recent years, Z has gone beyond the 26point2 distance to compete in ultra (and ultra-ultra) long categories. This increase in mileage has had a notable effect on his diet. He is now so used to extremely long distances that, "If the training is shorter than 20 km [12 miles], I don't eat during it. On longer distances, I take some energy bars or even better, oatmeal bars [he's partial to Davina Energy Oat Snacks and the oatmeal versions of CLIF bars]. After a longer training, I'll have a protein shake or high-protein meal such as meat, eggs, fresh cheese, beer (or tea in wintertime), and an isotonic drink."

3. What is your special, secret training tip?

Z says he has no special tips. I will say, in observation from the outside looking in, that having a highly active and large dog living in an urban apartment seems like great motivation to get frequent long runs in. Z's dog at one point needed hours of daily exercise, and so Z made it a habit to take Luna out to the great open areas and long paths that he knows so well. As a result, Z got in excellent training while his dog burned off some energy.

In the central area of Europe where Z is based, he also has easy access to spectacular mountain ranges and their surrounding foothills. He makes a point to take full advantage of the opportunity to train with the added running challenges that these landscapes provide. He's happy to do trail runs while plowing through knee-deep snow or trying to stay agile among thick mud puddles that crop up on the trails. Luna often joins in on the adventures as well.

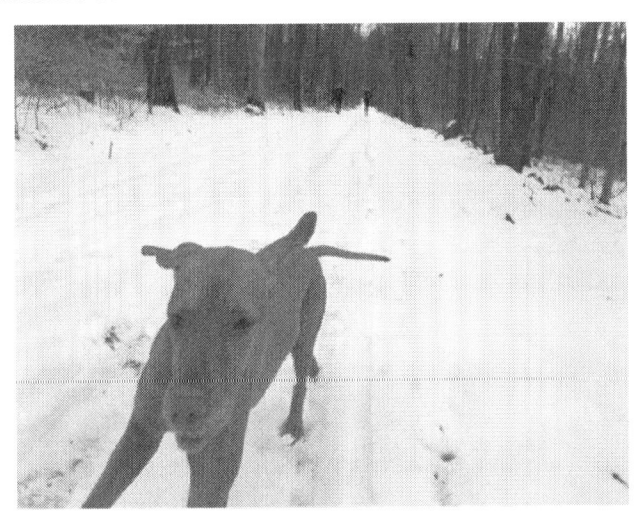

Luna on a snowy trail run. If you look closely, you can spot Z trailing behind (Photo courtesy of Z)

4. Is there any cultural influence, or something going on in your personal life, that impacts your training?

"In Croatia, when I was training with my local club, we always went to have a beer and hang out together outside of training." Having a close social network of runners undoubtedly contributes to the overall experience, and these groups seem to evolve organically in laid-back cultures such as Croatia.

5. Do you add any other exercise to your marathon preparation for cross training?

"After a few years of doing marathons, I started to do triathlons because I had the feeling that repeated monotonous running workouts could lead to injury. I think that involving other sports has been beneficial." What Z does not mention is the extreme endurance needed for the triathlons he chooses. He has successfully completed a double Ironman-length ultra-triathlon (swimming 4.8 miles (7.8 km), cycling 224 miles (360 km), and running 52.4 miles — a double marathon (84 km)). Z, we salute you!

6. How long is your marathon training cycle?

"For my first marathon, I had approximately six months (after I ran a half marathon). My personal philosophy is that a marathon equals three half marathons, not from a distance perspective, but in terms of effort. So, **I give my tendons and joints enough time to adjust to the long training sessions that are necessary for a marathon**."

Z went on to say that after his first two marathons, he no longer does a specific marathon training cycle, but rather tries to consistently be in good shape. This is in case he wants to sign up impulsively for a marathon (or longer ultra-marathon distance). He simply adds longer runs of about 33km (20 miles) a month or two before the race. "I like running so much that I want to be ready to do a major distance at any time."

7. What do you eat for breakfast on the day of your marathon?

"Usually I eat a pastry or roll, and I'll have some sliced sausage and cheese, or jam."

8. What did you eat and drink during the race? At what intervals?

Z relies on what is provided by the race organization for his race day fueling. "I take whatever is offered at refreshment points. So, water at the beginning, and later isotonic or cola beverages. I also like oranges a lot and watermelon, if available. Some salty snacks are also more than welcome." The only thing he might add to what's offered is his own supply of energy gels that he carries with him.

9. Deep thoughts: what was your mental preparation and focus throughout training and on race day? Do you use any outside running "distractions" (such as music, podcasts, running

apps, etc.) while running?

"I don't have any kind of special mental preparation. If I really care about the finish time, then I prepare a strategy for the speed I will run, but my mental focus is usually only on the city that I am running in, in order to soak up the environment." Z's preferred way to take the pulse of any new city is to explore it running.

"I started to run with music, but I quickly discovered that this was a "fun killer" like watching TV without sound or eating a cold burger while drinking a warm beer. Running without hearing the sounds around you, especially in nature, is just half of the experience. It can also distract you at a time when you should 'meet yourself,' although I can understand that some people are afraid of 'meeting themselves' and are intimidated by silence." For Z, not taking the opportunity to reflect with himself would lessen the impact of the experience.

***

"Methinks that the moment my legs began to move, my thoughts began to flow."

–Henry David Thoreau

***

10. What does your post-race period look like, both for recovery and celebrating? (Note: The celebration after crossing the finish line can serve as motivation that gets you through training and the race!)

Z says, "Very often after the race I go sight-seeing, but it would be smart to have a massage and rest."

Bonus Question: What should you NOT have done in your 26point2?

"Training is a good time to experiment, to try new equipment, or food and drink, and to change your routine. But **during the race, always do what you normally do, otherwise you may have some unwanted surprises**." This solid, tried-and-true advice is volleyed around time and time again for a reason. It seems simple, but in every race you always hear of some runner that, on impulse, tries out something new on race day and gets unpleasant results.

Z chooses to be surprised in other ways on race day. He namely enjoys feeling taken aback by unexpected scenery. Due to all the experience he has garnered, he prefers to over-prepare for his runs, both mentally and physically. That's why he does long distance trail runs to train for a marathon, all the while telling himself that he needs to be ready mentally to do the equivalent of "three half-marathon" races to successfully navigate his 26point2. That way, when race day rolls around, he can immerse himself in the environment, and fully engage in that in-depth one-on-one conversation with himself.

***

Željko Š., from Croatia, has run in Croatia, Austria, the Czech Republic, France, Germany, Hungary, Italy, Macedonia, Montenegro, Portugal, Russia, Serbia, Slovakia, and Slovenia

Mile 22: For the Love of Running

Diana D. from Latvia

At a pivotal moment in life, Latvian Diana D. destroyed one habit by picking up another. Upon returning to Europe after living an island lifestyle in the Maldives, she found herself gaining weight and frequently smoking. Diana felt a strong urge to improve the habits negatively affecting her health. She wanted to be more active and beat her addiction to cigarettes. Since Diana has a busy schedule, she felt that the least complicated way to start exercising was to throw on a pair of running shoes and go for a run. Through her training, Diane discovered that she had an incredible talent for distance running and embraced a newfound love for the sport.

Diana takes things to the extreme in her athletics. Once she triumphed at the 26point2 distance, she went on to achieve podium appearances at trail ultra-marathons around Europe. This drive carried over to other kinds of exercise, and when she started a yoga practice, this athletic aggrandizer was drawn to Bikram hot yoga to increase the intensity. In an attempt to stay loose and avoid injury, Diane made yoga the focal point of her stretching routine. In Bikram yoga, that stretching takes place in studios that are heated between 95–108 degrees Fahrenheit (35–42 Celsius).

The essence of running is a repeated back and forth motion that can shorten muscles over time due to constant tension. Yoga lengthens those same muscles and unlocks the tightness that accumulates. Adding heat to a yoga practice allows for deeper stretching, and a complete state of relaxation follows. Diana values this and now tries not to miss her weekly 90-minute sessions. Since her winter training takes place in quite cold conditions, it's an added bonus to do yoga in a hot and humid environment that leaves participants sweating instead of shivering. For Diana, swapping smoke for steam proved to be beneficial.

1. What time of day do you run and why?

"I run mostly early in the morning, at 5:00 a.m. I'm a single mother, and I need to find the best way to use my time for exercise that allows me to have more time to spend with my daughter."

2. What do you typically eat before or after training sessions?

Diana only fuels for running if she is going longer than 1.5 hours. If she's going out that long, she'll opt for the ever-popular energy bar and banana combo. After running, she'll eat a balanced meal such as eggs with porridge. "But if I have no time, I'll swap that for a protein shake instead."

3. What is your special, secret training tip?

"Just listen to your body," says Diana. This is a skill that she strengthens though her weekly hot yoga where the environment promotes a strong mind-body connection.

4. Is there any cultural influence, or something going on in your personal life, that impacts your training?

Early on, weight loss was a key motivation for Diana's running. After losing the weight, she said that the real reason she sticks with running (and gets incredible results) is because she feels genuine love for the sport. This goes in tandem with what author Christopher McDougall wrote about runners of the Tarahumara tribe from the Copper Canyon area of Mexico.

Claims have been made that lifestyle components of the Tarahumara, such as diet and the infrastructure of their homeland, make them the phenomenal super athletes that they are. In his book *Born to Run*, the author best describes the true essence of their running when he says, "That was the real secret of the Tarahumara: they'd never forgotten what it felt like to love running…And like everything else we love — everything we sentimentally call our 'passions' and 'desires' it's really an encoded ancestral necessity. We were born to run; we were born because we run. We're all Running People, as the Tarahumara have always known." Diana also runs her best when she feels that deeply rooted joy for running. "You can be successful only if you really enjoy what you do," she enthuses.

5. Do you add any other exercise to your marathon preparation for cross training?

Beyond yoga, Diana swims. "I'm confident that these two things help me to avoid injuries…since I've been doing them, I don't have any complaints of anything hurting."

6. How long is your marathon training cycle?

Diana feels that a twelve-week training cycle is the ideal amount of time to get prepared and build endurance to avoid injuries.

7. What do you eat for breakfast on the day of your marathon?

Diana's portable and practical breakfast consisting of carbs, sugar, fat, and protein could be taken straight out of an elementary school lunch box from the USA. She loves peanut butter and jelly sandwiches, and before a marathon she will eat one or two with a banana as well. This easily portable option is ideal for taking along to destination races.

8. What did you eat and drink during the race? At what intervals?

"I take one gel every 8 km [5 miles], and I drink water after taking it. I have figured out that this is the best way to prevent me from getting low on sugar and feeling weak. I don't eat any other food during the race. I will have cola once or twice over the last 15 km [9 miles] if available."

9. Deep thoughts: what was your mental preparation and focus throughout training and on race day? Do you use any outside running "distractions" (such as music, podcasts, running apps, etc.) while running?

"During training, what helps me the most is to visualize myself crossing the finish line feeling that adrenaline rush of achieving my goal." But during the race, Diana takes a different approach. "I do not think of reaching the finish line at all. I just listen to music and just keep pushing forward without concentrating too hard on anything."

10. What does your post-race period look like, both for recovery and celebrating? (Note: The celebration after crossing the finish line can serve as motivation that gets you through training and the race!)

"After the race, I am happy to eat as much as I want of anything I'm in the mood for. Then I let my body rest and enjoy the feeling of doing absolutely nothing."

As she races around Europe, Diana notes with appreciation that, "At all the races I've been in, there have been such nice people at the aid stations. They always seem amazed by us runners, and this is what I love so much. They look up to you like you are a hero, and I feel I get extra support because there are fewer women participants."

Diana feels that love and channels it towards her own positive feelings about running to reach her impressive goals.

***

**Diana D., from Latvia, has run in
Latvia, Austria, Estonia, France, and Iceland**

Mile 23: Intentional Running

Peter H. From Australia

Training for a marathon, much like life itself, comes with inevitable highs and lows. Some lows actually feel like rock bottom, but in the training process, moving forward can be uplifting and become part of the solution. Peter H. has experienced some of the biggest challenges that life can throw at you. Although he is from Australia and the places where he runs boast impressively beautiful scenery, people also struggle in paradise. By means of Peter's hard work and dedicated training, serene living and running success have prevailed.

Peter puts in an extraordinary amount of effort to make his endurance training a lifestyle. This is apparent not only when his running shoes are laced up but throughout many other aspects of his life. He puts in a lot of time to do challenging training sessions — including frequent strength-building work with weights — and makes getting an ideal amount of rest a top priority. He turns to fresh produce for refueling and will add a decidedly Aussie touch to his diet in the form of a dark yeasty paste. All of these components help Peter sustain balance and avoid letting difficult moments weigh him down.

1. What time of day do you run and why?

"In a perfect world, I would run mid-morning!" Peter declares. Yet, as we all know, real life (including work and responsibilities) often derails our perfect training scenarios. So, Peter defers to evening runs and often alters his morning preference on the weekend to more closely match race day conditions. "I like to go for a long run in the middle of the day on the weekend. This is to ensure I am getting the effects of the full heat of the day in case I face hot conditions on race day."

2. What do you typically eat before or after training sessions?

Peter ensures he has a fresh cold-pressed juice waiting for him when he returns from long workouts. "Natural sugar and cold. Yum!!! And since they are liquid, they quickly restore what has just been used." Taking the time to leave yourself a refreshing and natural pick-me-up incorporates self-care into the marathon training process. Living in a county such as Australia, where incredible seasonal produce is widely available, make juicing a no-brainer.

3. What is your special, secret training tip?

"Get a coach!! The accountability of answering to someone and having someone there for you is priceless. I wish I had done this years ago…If you are trying to get to the next level this is the key!"

A coach takes the guesswork out of the best marathon training for individual situations and goals. There are also many different forms of coaching available, so it doesn't have to cost a fortune. As seen in Chapter 19 with Iván, group sessions with a coach provide accountability and guidance, but the costs are split up among the members. Julio M.C. from Chapter 11 offers long-distance coaching via the internet. This option provides curated information and a plan of action shaped to reach specific objectives. Additionally, as Julio employs the shared workout function on the Strava app in his coaching, it forces the runner to stay honest about the work put in.

Another marathoner equated having a coach to counting on a highly informed running pal on call for reassurance about specific issues. For example, this person was training hard with a clear focus of hitting a Boston Marathon qualification time. As part of this plan, she took her speed workouts very seriously. When some running friends were traveling to a nearby town to do a fun 10K road race, she felt torn. She didn't know if that distance would throw a wrench in her prescribed workout. After a quick consultation with her coach, she made the recommended adjustments for that week's training and was able to enjoy the 10K without any worry. A coach can take varying components of a workout plan and mix together the winning formula while providing a sounding board for all running-related doubts.

4. Is there any cultural influence, or something going on in your personal life, that impacts your training?

Here Peter shares a personal story about the deeply positive influence that training has had on his life. "After a 15-year battle with drugs, I needed a replacement and endurance sport was the answer. I have an addictive personality…for me, it's all or nothing. So, I made sports my habit."

Despite his intense relationship with running, moderation in everything in life, even healthy activities, is best. Peter recognizes this. The level of focus he dedicates to training demands that he places equally high attention on restoration and rest. To do this, Peter lives the dream…by dreaming. His key for recovery is to, "Sleep and sleep and sleep, at least eight to nine hours minimum every night."

It seems counterintuitive, but resting so well takes incredible effort. This is because you need real dedication to stop doing whatever else keeps you up late. Many of us are short on sleep and haven't yet found the way to cut out less meaningful activities, such as zoning out with Netflix or scrolling through Instagram, and actually get into bed. But adequate rest is crucial for success, and Peter makes it a priority to get it.

5. Do you add any other exercise to your marathon preparation for cross training?

According to Peter, "Core strength is the key!!! I cannot stress enough how crucial weights are! I always allow for at least three sessions of weightlifting per week. I know running is a lean sport, but tailoring a strength-training program to gain core strength is important." Many runners have a preference for cardio cross training, but the time spent in the weight room working on a strong core translates to better running posture and therefore improved efficiency.

6. How long is your marathon training cycle?

For Peter, the answer here depends entirely on what goals he's trying to achieve. With each race, he'll consider his objectives and collaborate with his coach on a timeline that will best help to reach (or surpass!) them.

7. What do you eat for breakfast on the day of your marathon?

"Oats that have already fully absorbed milk for a mix of protein and carbs, finished with one piece of toast, no butter but Vegemite for the salty factor. I wash it all down with a double espresso and a hydration drink."

There seems to be a continental divide over the best toast spreads ranging from peanut butter to olive oil to Marmite, with Vegemite as the top contender from Australia. Vegemite is the beloved version of Marmite that was created in wartime when access to products from the UK was limited. Some say there is a distinctly more "veggie" taste in Vegemite (hence the name) yet both products have a similar consistency and umami-based flavor that runners in these parts of the world crave.

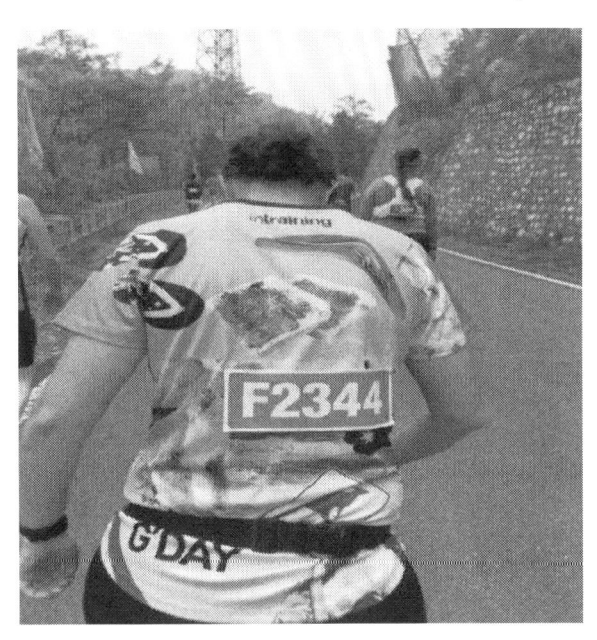

An Australian runner puts her love of Vegemite on proud display at a destination marathon (Photo: M.A. Nixon)

8. What did you eat and drink during the race? At what intervals?

"I use gels and think the High5Plus [www.high5.co.uk] line is excellent. As far as frequency, just be sure to train with what you race with. You must **play around and learn what works for you here, as we are all different.**"

9. Deep thoughts: what was your mental preparation and focus throughout training and on race day? Do you use any outside running "distractions" (such as music, podcasts, running apps, etc.) while running?

In Peter's opinion, many people don't fully recognize the mental component involved in distance running. "People that are not driven, or not into an endurance sport, do not understand this. Mental toughness and self-doubt crawl into your training and preparation. Every day and each session involve a mental fight. I find I can go from self-doubt to glory, to doubting to finishing all within a single run. This sport is a mental roller coaster."

Knowing that these feelings can arise is the first step in finding a formula to overcome them. To fight back against the negativity, Peter shows up strong, hydrated, fueled, and well-rested and gives his all. He knows he can push through the tough moments and that positivity and serene feelings will follow.

10. What does your post-race period look like, both for recovery and celebrating? (Note: The celebration after crossing the finish line can serve as motivation that gets you through training and the race!)

"Definitely a massage and sleep...but when you work that hard you deserve to party, too!"

There's no doubt that training and race day evoke a wide range of feelings. Many runners get emotional after crossing the finish line of a 26point2 because of all the hard work, tightly interwoven with high and low moments, that is involved with reaching the goal. A marathon is both a physical and mental journey requiring preparation of body and mind. There can be very rough moments during a marathon where the best option seems to be giving up. Even while running in some of the most amazing natural beauty on Earth, Peter also feels the lows. But both in his running and his life, he always finds a way to move forward and persevere. Good on ya, mate!

***

Peter H., from Australia, has run in Australia

Mile 24: Run the World
Becky W. from USA

Becky W. is Becky Wade. This elite runner requires a complete introduction so that we can all cheer her on in the Olympic Games where, if things roll out as envisioned, the runner named "America's best young marathoner" by Runner's World magazine will represent the United States! Becky's professional running career is still in its infancy, so the best is likely yet to come. However, we can all anticipate outstanding achievements from this already accomplished athlete.

While researching my dream running destination, the famed Yaya Village training camp in Ethiopia, I came across Becky's profile as one of the camp's international ambassadors. Established in collaboration with beloved Ethiopian running champ Haile Gebrselassie, the Yaya Village holds its mission to be "A world-class high-altitude training facility for both local and international endurance athletes." A stay at the village to train provides a cultural exchange among international and local Ethiopian runners that is both meaningful and beneficial.

Becky's time in Ethiopia was spent learning how the local runners, who are some of the strongest distance runners in the world, train and race. It was a rewarding stay, and she has stated that she hopes to visit yearly and make the Yaya Village her high-altitude training base. She first came across this singular experience as she was organizing another singular experience: a year-long exploratory running trip around the world.

Besides being a highly decorated elite athlete that won the very first marathon in which she ever participated, Becky is an avid international traveler. She shares that she came across the Yaya Village as part of a year-long epic journey in which she set out to study, "Foreign running communities, searching for both unique and common ways that people around the world approach running and construct their lives around it." She was able to carry out this dream trip by securing a fellowship that funded her experience; writing a book was the subsequent result of her findings while traveling the globe and connecting with international runners along the way.

Galvanized by her adventure after exploring nine different running cultures all over the world, Becky documented the experiences in a book called *Run the World*. Here, she puts on her storytelling hat and describes her highly varied running experiences as she was hosted in a total of 72 homes around the world. She connected with so many people from widely varying cultures through a shared love of running. In doing so, she was able to apply some of what she learned to her own elite routine. Becky is *Around the Globe in 26point2 Miles* personified.

For a direct look at Becky's multi-country running adventure, including the array of food that other runners from around the world lovingly prepared for her training (she shared the recipes!), the strategies she used to discover prime running spots in new places, the culturally based recovery methods she tried, and the connections forged with other runners, you can go to www.harpercollins.com and order *Run the World*. Anyone who has raced outside of their own zip code will connect with Becky's experiences. To learn how an elite marathoner put new knowledge into practice in order to get exceptional results, see Becky's nuanced insight below.

1. What time of day do you run and why?

Becky's main running session is always first thing in the morning. She is an early riser and feels most alert around daybreak. As an elite pro athlete, she often incorporates a second run after doing different kinds of workouts. She finds closure in rounding out the day by having her final run coincide with the sunset. She saves her stretching and foam rolling for before bedtime, which makes great sense.

Foam rolling, or self-myofascial release, as trainers, pros, and physical therapists call it, is an effective and relaxing tension release practice that can be done after a run. By using your own weight on top of a foam roller and rolling, the back and forth movement helps to free up muscular tight spots and promote blood flow. The technique has been applauded for achieving optimal muscle and tissue health, and, beyond that, it is incredibly relaxing and promotes an overall sense of well-being. I always feel lighter, taller, and slightly euphoric after a good rolling session. Once you start the practice after a tough workout, you'll never look back and will quite possibly find yourself, as I do, taking your roller with you everywhere, even on vacation.

Throughout the day the body becomes compacted and tense, therefore saving a stretching and foam rolling session for later in the evening, as Becky does, delivers advantages. As each step taken (or run) adds to compression, rolling out the major muscles and the spine provides excellent release from the tension. The practice will leave you calmer and more relaxed for sleeping as well.

2. What do you typically eat before or after training sessions?

"I always eat a bagel with peanut butter, banana, and honey before my long runs and big workouts (assuming I have 2.5–3.5 hours to digest). I fuel mid-run with Sword and refuel with a CLIF bar or fruit and a protein smoothie." Sword energy drinks (www.drinksword.com) are popular with elite athletes and are said to delay fatigue without causing an upset stomach.

3. What is your special, secret training tip?

There are no secrets here because in interviews, the articles she pens, her blog, and on social media, there are innumerable helpful tips and tweaks that Becky happily shares. Her ideas help runners streamline their nutrition, dress thoughtfully for all kinds of weather, and get better rest. For example, a simple tip that Becky shared in an interview solved a situation that I had been struggling with until she brought an uncomplicated solution to my attention. Becky frequently adds smoothies to her training diet. She even reps for a new line of smoothie filled CLIF bars that are said to be delicious.

I also like to make smoothies, but with some recipes, getting the quantities just right was a challenge. I'd gather the ingredients for my favorite green smoothie (consisting of lemon, apple, banana, pear, spinach, arugula, and celery) and after making one, there'd inevitably be odd amounts of leftover ingredients that would quickly spoil. I didn't like making big batches, however, since the banana ingredient often turned the whole drink brown within hours. The process seemed wasteful, and I started to make fewer smoothies.

Then I learned that Becky portions out her extra smoothie leftovers and immediately freezes them. She takes a serving out of the freezer before her run, and by the time she finishes, they are ready to be consumed and still nice and cold. I've tried it with my green smoothie recipe and can confirm that the individual portions are delicious, convenient and avoid the unappealing brown banana effect.

Additionally, Becky trains in the mountains of Colorado where days with sunny blue skies and fluffy clouds can be deceptively bitter cold. She realizes that her core and legs eventually warm up during her workouts while her extremities can remain chilled. She combats this issue with what she calls "confused ensembles" entailing sports bras and tiny running shorts paired with gloves and compression sleeves. She pokes fun at her unusual but practical outfits in her Instagram feed with emojis of bikinis and furry mittens. Becky wears what works for her running regardless of the fashion statement she may or may not be making.

Lastly, Becky doled out tips in a recent article that she

wrote for Runner's World magazine, where she shared that she struggles seriously with insomnia. She realizes the significant role that quality sleep plays in optimal running performance, so she thought it was helpful to open up about this personal issue and share her wisdom on the topic.

In her piece entitled *I'm an Elite Marathoner with Sleep Issues. Here's How I Manage Them*, Becky names the things she requires to increase her chances of a good night's sleep, including, "Going to bed at a consistent time, reading until my eyelids droop, keeping my bedroom chilly, shedding my watch, eating a small snack, using all the suggested tools (blackout curtains, earplugs, eye mask, and white noise machine), and relaxing before bedtime. I'm a fan of light-hearted shows (think *The Office* and *The Great British Bake Off*), gentle stretching, hot baths, and books that are engaging but not unsettling." These are all good pointers that can often be overlooked. I find it especially easy to forget to shed my watch (or remove my phone from the bedroom), and if I wake up in the night and see the time, it's definitely not conducive to good sleep.

4. Is there any cultural influence, or something going on in your personal life, that impacts your training?

Becky had a key takeaway from her time in Ethiopia. "The biggest cultural impact on my training was the ability of Ethiopian runners to go with the flow, follow the leader, and not worry about controlling all of the variables (time, pace, distance, etc.)." Since Becky was so accustomed to diligently following structured running plans under coaches, this was a fresh approach for her and allowed her to experience her running in a free and joyous way.

5. Do you add any other exercise to your marathon preparation for cross training?

"I do a general strength routine after my hard workouts (usually twice a week), which is mostly body weight work and takes about 30 minutes. I do a core circuit about 5 times a week."

6. How long is your marathon training cycle?

"My marathon cycles tend to be 12–16 weeks. For me, this amount of time seems to be long enough to get in very good shape but not so long that I'm burned out by the end."

7. What do you eat for breakfast on the day of your marathon?

Becky has access to top coaches and nutritionists to guide her fueling, and she has learned over the years of her career what works best for her. "I eat the same thing before races as I do for workouts so I don't have to worry about how my body will respond. I just love the peanut butter and banana combo and find it to be very satiating."

8. What did you eat and drink during the race? At what intervals?

Elite runners have water bottles waiting for them on tables at exactly every 5 km marking point throughout the race. While this knowledge might be filed under "Information I will never need to take advantage of," since this is not my racing category, I could look at it in a different way. If the elites are doing it, it must be for a good, results-based reason! Replicating this strategy to rehydrate every 3 miles (5 km) is a helpful guideline for optimal performance. If upon studying the racecourse you realize that there are aid stations spaced further than 5 km apart, you may want to involve a supportive person to be stationed closer with your own personal hydration or fueling options. For these purposes, Becky again turns to her beverage of choice, Sword performance drink. "I take a few big gulps of Sword every 5 km during a marathon. That's how often elite bottles are set out, and that's what I train to do."

9. Deep thoughts: what was your mental preparation and focus throughout training and on race day? Do you use any outside running "distractions" (such as music, podcasts, running

apps, etc.) while running?

"My mental prep happens every day in training and is something I've been honing for years. I break down a race into manageable chunks, I try to stay present, and I try to use the momentum offered by the crowd and my competitors."

Chunking any endeavor into manageable portions instead of one big undertaking is wise. During a low moment mid-race, for example, it feels less daunting to center your thoughts on getting through the current mile, rather than focusing on the total remaining. Once that manageable smaller goal is achieved, your perspective will be buoyed, and you'll feel more positive.

Becky also emphasized that she thrives from crowd support during her 26point2. While this is not a factor that can be counted on in many smaller marathons held in less-populated areas around the world, in big races in major cities you can likely count on this frenetic energy to spur on your efforts.

I can only imagine what Becky's typical situation must feel like. She is usually cheered on as the first runner heading the lead marathon pack. Countless fans know her story and cheer her on by name. As a leading female runner in most races, Becky not only gets frenzied cheers from everybody lining the racecourse, she also gets specific updates and detailed information on where the other contenders stand in relation to her and how they are performing. Additionally, her support team shouts out feedback on her form as she flies by, so she can make improvements as needed.

What we mere mortals can take away from Becky's experiences is that it could be a really positive thing to have an informed person or two in the crowd looking out for you during your 26point2. If that person knows your running style and can identify things for you to work on, such as incorporating your arms more or improving your posture, you will have a distinct advantage. When I start to feel very worn down mid-race, just deciding on what to focus on seems to take too much effort. I sometimes feel like a puppet during a race, and when people offer up helpful feedback, they pull my strings in the right direction.

10. What does your post-race period look like, both for recovery and celebrating? (Note: The celebration after crossing the finish line can serve as motivation that gets you through training and the race!)

"After each marathon, I get a flush-out massage within a couple days of racing, I do a super light jog the next day to assess the state of my body, and I eat whatever I'm craving for the week or so after. I usually celebrate with the members of my support team (coach, husband, parents, siblings, etc.) with a good meal and a few drinks."

Becky chose to skip the bonus question about what NOT to do on race day. For her, it is expendable. Even her very first marathon experience was a wild success due to nothing less than the meticulous care taken towards all the details of her running. This, along with her sharp focus and diligence, has brought her to the top of the podium on that run and on a multitude of occasions.

With major running aspirations in the pipeline, Becky has stated what all marathoners know deep down: "There are so many variables on race day, and it's hard to nail them all on the same day." While this is undeniably true, when you run the world, you can identify what works for you and what doesn't, and act accordingly.

***

Becky W., from USA, has run in USA, Australia, Denmark, England, Ethiopia, Finland, France, Ireland, Italy, Japan, New Zealand, Poland, South Korea, Spain, Sweden, and Switzerland

Around the Globe in 26point2 Miles

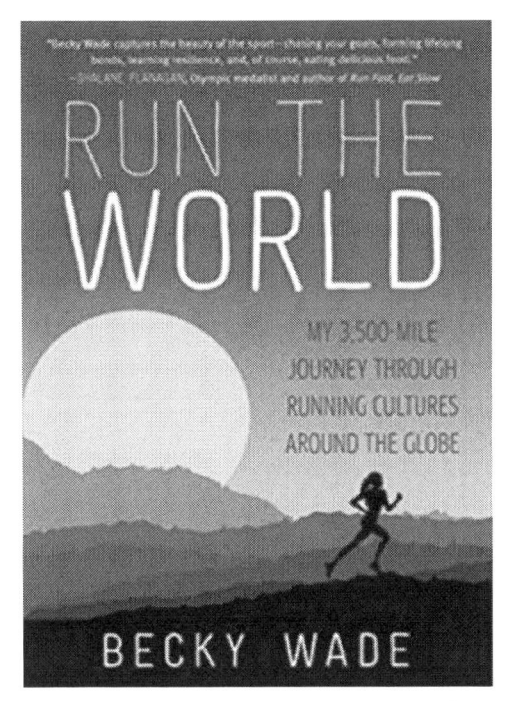

Becky Wade's globetrotting adventure Run the World

Mile 25: Compression and Decompression

Emmanuelle G. from France

Emmanuelle G. approaches her marathon training with the same commitment and competency that landed top-level roles in her career in finance well before she turned 30. When traveling the globe for professional purposes or living abroad for work (as she's done in four different countries), this French runner seamlessly blends her two worlds.

Emmanuelle thrives on success and works well in new and challenging situations. This was apparent when she merged a destination marathon with the beginning segment of a work trip. Her post-26point2 celebratory meal consisted of wine and hors d'oeuvres at a business cocktail reception she took part in just hours after crossing the finish line. She was able to evoke her Parisian sheen and swiftly change from running shoes to high-powered executive heels to attend the event.

In retrospect, though, she says the next time she will plan that particular sequence a bit differently and add a bit more food to the equation. "I was so hungry after my race, and only 'flying finger food' on circulating trays was available at my work event. It was my mistake; next time I won't wait, and I'll arrange my own food-focused celebration immediately after the race."

While she recognizes that it's a challenge to go on business trips during a crucial point of a training cycle, Emmanuelle focuses on the positive aspects of her preferred sport. "**Running is the one sport I can always train for when traveling. I can run in any weather, on any surface, and at any time**. It's pretty much the most flexible sport in the world."

No matter where she runs in the world, Emmanuelle looks to infuse her running experience with a long-standing French tradition. Without fail, there is a well-selected celebratory wine after her races; I've even waited for her under the Eiffel Tower with her lovely parents and an open bottle of excellent champagne to toast her immediately after finishing a Parisian race. In addition, she also tries when possible to combine her destination racing and training with all things wine-related. Emmanuelle runs in areas where she's able to visit family-run wineries, she participates in vineyard races, and she partakes in wine tasting events after running.

Emmanuelle's style is one of the first things people notice about her. How anyone can look so put together at a 7:00 a.m. training run is beyond me. "I'm never without my eyeliner, and it seems to hold well," she says. Additionally, her sleek trademark bun easily makes the transition from a trail run to a conference meeting room. She is the epitome of "French girl chic."

Yet Emmanuelle's running look goes beyond hair and makeup. When showing a photo of her running in a stunning vineyard to a non-runner friend, my friend's first comment to me was not about the scenery. "Break down her outfit to me, I don't understand what she's wearing," she said. This was because Emmanuelle often wears long compression socks and sleeves. These accessories are beneficial to runners, or anyone working out outdoors, as the light pressure applied by the snug-fitting socks or removable sleeves aid with circulation and blood flow.

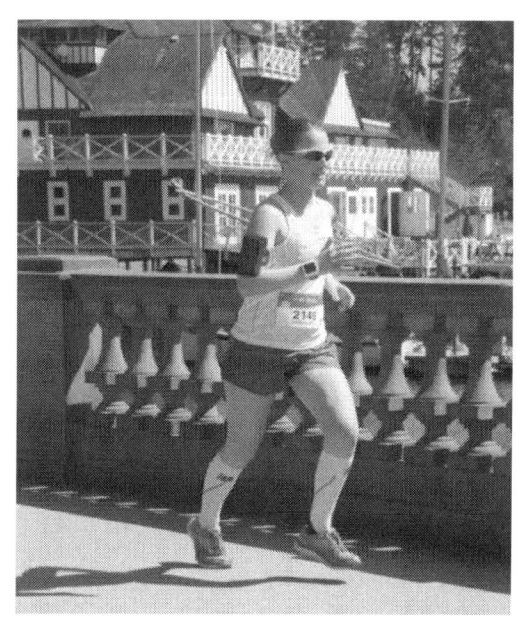

Emmanuelle — and her compression socks — on the run. Allez, allez! (Photo courtesy of Emmanuelle)

For Emmanuelle, however, they serve a more practical purpose for her training, especially when she gets out of the city. "I appreciate them on trails because they protect me a bit from scratches when running too close to brambles or branches. I also use these when the weather shifts and long sleeves are too much, but short sleeves are a little chilly. They give me peace of mind in terms of feeling comfortable at any temperature."

The multipurpose sleeves and socks provide warmth, protection, and a bit of light compression all wrapped up in a single running accessory. For Emmanuelle, the perfect pairing for any compression is a little decompression after her running in the form of some freshly uncorked bottles of wine for sampling.

1. What time of day do you run and why?

Emmanuelle adds flexibility to her running schedule and changes times according to the training she aims to do. "For short easy runs (6–8 km [3.5–5 miles]), I prefer early morning (pre-breakfast), at a slow pace. For intervals and tempo mid-distance (9–14 km [5–9 miles]), I prefer late morning or afternoon as I have more energy and power to push through the intensity. For long-distance runs, on the weekend, I like to go out mid-morning, usually about one hour after breakfast."

2. What do you typically eat before or after training sessions?

During a long run or a mid-distance tempo run, Emmanuelle will have a few gummy power shots (from the PowerBar brand) and/or a gel (she opts for the GU brand).

3. What is your special, secret training tip?

"Planning, planning, planning," is critical Emmanuelle says, but she also emphasizes that it's important not to push too hard with overly ambitious training plans. "I actually pushed too hard in training and arrived tired on race day once." A tapering down period starting about ten days to two weeks before race day is ideal to show up rested and ready at the starting line.

4. Is there any cultural influence, or something going on in your personal life, that impacts your training?

"I had a last-minute business trip to Kazakhstan... which nearly destroyed my entire week of marathon training due to jetlag." Emmanuelle coped with this by pushing herself to go out into the bitterly cold mornings (-13 degrees Fahrenheit (-25 degrees Celsius)) to explore the area and get some fresh air. She was grateful for these exhilarating runs as they energized her muddled jetlag mornings and allowed her to explore Astana as she spent the rest of her time in Kazakhstan indoors in meetings.

5. Do you add any other exercise to your marathon preparation for cross training?

Emmanuelle is happy to overlap her marathon training into the sphere of triathlon workouts and will gladly add in swimming one or two times a week and spinning at least once a week. She looks to vary her workouts so she can utilize different muscle groups while still getting in aerobic activity.

6. How long is your marathon training cycle?

As Emmanuelle is generally in top shape, she feels ready to suit up for a marathon with eight weeks' notice or less.

7. What do you eat for breakfast on the day of your marathon?

"I eat plain yogurt and a banana with a cup of coffee, and about 40 minutes before starting I have an isotonic drink with an energy bar," simply because, "I always eat that before a race."

8. What did you eat and drink during the race? At what intervals?

Emmanuelle drinks water, and she'll alternate the previously mentioned gummies she eats at the 10-20-30-km marks with gels taken at the 15-25-35-40-km points.

9. Deep thoughts: what was your mental preparation and focus throughout training and on race day? Do you use any outside running "distractions" (such as music, podcasts, running apps, etc.) while running?

Here, Emmanuelle simply states that she finds it helpful to "mostly run with music."

10. What does your post-race period look like, both for recovery and celebrating? (Note: The celebration after crossing the finish line can serve as motivation that gets you through training and the race!)

The one thing that Emmanuelle always looks forward to after reaching the finish line is a simple post-marathon indulgence: a long, hot shower.

With her well-honed decompression techniques, it is also guaranteed that from Iceland to Tahiti she'll find some excellent wine to uncork for her celebration!

***

Emmanuelle G., from France, has run in France, Austria, Canada, the Czech Republic, Estonia, Iceland, Italy, Kazakhstan, South Korea, Spain, Switzerland, Tahiti, the UK, and USA

Mile 26: My 26point2

Mary Anne N. from USA

My background story is provided in the introduction, so I'll jump right into the questions.

1. What time of day do you run and why?

Morning training sessions work best for me during marathon preparation. Life in Sevilla is full of spontaneous meetups and last-minute plans. You may bump into a long-lost friend on your way home from the market and have a leisurely coffee to catch up, or you might hear about a flamenco concert just minutes before it begins. I felt the need to do my workouts early because I found that if I didn't, something would inevitably come up and derail even my best intentions.

For subsequent marathons a few years later, I had a whole new spontaneous element to organize training runs around: a new baby in the house! Trying to get out for long weekend workouts now meant that there were many more factors that needed to correctly fall into place, including how the baby was doing that day, if she'd slept the night before, and childcare logistics. I once again found that getting the runs in early in the day was an effective strategy to increase the odds of successful training. If it was impossible to get out early in the morning, there was still hope for an evening run later on.

2. What do you typically eat before or after training sessions?

My answer here is quite simple and straightforward: bananas, bananas, and more bananas. I tried to eat a banana before each and every run, in various shapes and forms. Banana smoothies are my favorite, while two-ingredient banana pancakes (just beat an egg together with a smashed banana and cook on the griddle) and banana bread muffins are also in my breakfast rotation.

Also, to be fully honest, my training diet consisted of a considerable amount of cheese, olives, and red *Ribera del Duero* wine, because I was living in Spain, and these things were part of daily life that I embraced. I'm not one of those people that drastically change their entire diet for marathon preparation. I always try to eat a generally healthy and clean diet and was just a bit more focused on eating well during the 10 weeks leading up to the marathon. I did, however, try to avoid consuming large amounts of alcohol on the nights before my long Sunday runs and of course the night before race day.

3. What is your special, secret training tip?

Sports massage therapy is extremely helpful for recovery after long runs and also serves as a way to keep track of the progress of recurring running injuries. My running friends refer to this as "vehicle maintenance," and I have to say I agree with this amusing parallel. I wouldn't take a 40-year-old car on a major road trip without a tune-up, so why not treat my 40-year-old body with the same care? For me, getting pre-marathon "tune-ups" is essential for wellbeing and helps to avoid injury-related complications during training.

4. Is there any cultural influence, or something going on in your personal life, that impacts your training?

Absolutely! The culture of Sevilla, Spain, where I lived impacted many aspects of my training experience. Sevilla is a very social city. There is a warm and inclusive cultural climate, especially when a shared interest is involved. Within the fabric of this vibrant city, there is room for foreigners to be woven in.

In Sevilla, I was fortunate enough to stumble across a running club that impacted my life and my perspective towards the sport. The name of the club is *Los Jartibles*, which roughly translates to "Those Who Can Never Get Enough." Those runners, who formed the core of my marathon training group, became a second family to me. Incidentally, the group also lives up to its cheeky name and can never get enough of unique race experiences, post-run breakfasts (or beers), and all-night holiday parties. All gatherings include a dose, however big or small, of running.

I realize that running by its very nature has an element of solitary reflection and can provide an opportunity to become absorbed in deep thoughts or lost in music or a compelling podcast. However, the social aspect of *Los Jartibles* really clicked with me on another level, especially with the goal of the marathon looming on the horizon. Suddenly, among a tight-knit group of runners, the miles (kilometers on this side of the pond) flew by and *las tiradas largas* or Sunday morning long runs through the foggy olive groves became fun social adventures that made getting up before 7 a.m. on the weekend something to get excited about.

As we tackled these Sunday milestones weekly, spirited conversations ensued which were left unfinished before our three-hour running sessions came to an end. I love running, but highly doubted my own ability to maintain the discipline to run on my own, for that length of time, early morning in the middle of the countryside.

During the week, shorter 6:30 a.m. runs in the brisk and saturated winter air were doable on my own. Stretching and injury prevention through massage were also fine to manage on my own. Yet those long training runs in the Spanish countryside were infinitely better in the company of fun running buddies. It made a world of difference and absolutely contributed to the positive results I achieved with my PR marathon time.

There were also supportive spouses and friends of runners that would bike ahead on our routes, leave out water for us along the paths and even take pictures of us in action to provide memories of the whole marathon training process. (*Gra-*

cias Pepe!!)

5. Do you add any other exercise to your marathon preparation for cross training?

My running benefits from a regular yoga practice and I feel great when doing hot yoga. Ideally, I would go to Bikram yoga weekly but getting to a 90-minute class that often on top of marathon training just isn't my reality. Instead, I do smaller yoga sessions at home, with the added challenge of warding off my curious pup from doing her own downward dogs on my mat.

6. How long is your marathon training cycle?

I start working towards the marathon by slowly incorporating a few half marathons into my running program to increase my overall mileage. When I hit the "Ten weeks to go before race time" mark, I switch over to a more organized marathon preparation plan. Within the framework of that plan, I always account for the need to be flexible.

I find that the "race to train" strategy can keep things fresh and exciting during marathon preparation. If I know I need to do a 13-mile (21 km) run, I figure that it is more fun to do one in the form of a half marathon, with the energy of the other runners and the crowd to push me on. The routes are usually in new places where I don't typically run, so that keeps things interesting, and I feel committed to carrying out the training after registering for the race and paying for it in advance.

7. What do you eat for breakfast on the day of your marathon?

I was worried about running out of steam during my marathon, so I ate quite a bit more for breakfast on race day than most runners I know, but it worked for me and I felt great throughout the whole race. My morning meal consisted of coffee, one half of a gluten-free baguette with olive oil and sea salt, and a hunger-satiating walnut smoothie. The smoothie is a delicious caloric bomb that keeps me full for an entire morning due to the walnuts, dates, and Greek yogurt it contains. Genius food blogger Aida Mollenkamp created this recipe and it can be found at www.saltandwind.com.

Why gluten-free bread? I don't have issues with gluten, but I was told that it is linked to muscle inflammation, which is something to avoid before a big race. I didn't research the subject in depth, and I'm by no means an expert on the topic, so if you want more information on the effects of gluten, please contact a nutritionist. However, if advice doesn't seem too crazy and comes from a reliable source, I'm usually willing to try it out and so I avoided gluten before the race. I knew I still wanted to eat a carbohydrate-rich meal the night before, so I swapped out the traditional pasta dinner for a rice dish and devoured my lucky sweet potato oven fries instead.

The morning of my marathon, besides my giant breakfast, I also ate one banana and drank almost a liter of water. I ate the bigger meal 2.5 hours before the race, so as to not run with a full stomach, and saved the banana for about 15 minutes before the starting pistol went off, for a last boost of energy.

8. What did you eat and drink during the race? At what intervals?

During the race I drink plain old water, and occasionally sip on an isotonic drink when it's offered. I slip a few "emergency energy gels" into my waist pack with the intention of taking one about every hour but admittedly I don't usually do a great job of remembering to do so. I eat such a solid breakfast that I really don't feel the need for gels and have never finished a whole one. For the 26point2 distance, I find that gels serve as more of an insurance policy for me than anything else. I feel better knowing that I have them on me in case I start to fade, but I might not even use them.

9. Deep thoughts: what was your mental preparation and focus throughout training and on race day? Do you use any outside running "distractions" (such as music, podcasts, running

apps, etc.) while running?

To say that I am nervous the day of the race is an understatement; the energy running through me feels electric! However, I had a few small tricks up my sleeve to channel that energy and keep it high throughout the entire race.

I like to download a brand new, upbeat running playlist before a marathon. My trick involves the timing of when to use the new playlist. I love the atmosphere of a marathon, especially if music is also featured at various points along the course. My tweak, therefore, is to save the music for the home stretch. With about 45 minutes left to go, a curated playlist of high-energy songs provides a much-needed boost. By that point, music is uplifting and helps me cross the finish line.

At one 26point2, I was lucky enough to have a different focus as friends staggered themselves around the race route with awesome signs to cheer me on. Their support changed my nervous energy into an injection of positivity! It was truly amazing to see my name and motivating messages as I ran past. I highly recommend enlisting friends and family to provide personal support on race day. These kind souls should ideally distribute themselves along the marathon route instead of standing all in one place. The love and encouragement in the air the day I ran my marathon felt almost palpable. I even fed off the positive energy from other people's supporters, as their joy was contagious.

10. What does your post-race period look like, both for recovery and celebrating? (Note: The celebration after crossing the finish line can serve as motivation that gets you through training and the race!)

A post-race massage for total relaxation is great, but I like to wait a few days after the run to book one. Sevilla is home to an Arab bathhouse with a spa, where I had organized a post-marathon float in a unique and relaxing place. You can dip in pools of varying temperatures to loosen muscles, sip herbal tea in eucalyptus steam rooms, and get a wide array of spa services in an exotic environment. Knowing that such pampering is lined up after the race can serve as motivation while you run.

In a later marathon that I ran in the spa region of Slovenia, I discovered that a pool with jets of water at varying pressure points was an effective and gentle alternative to massage immediately after a marathon. You can position your muscles to get the water pressure to align with the especially stiff areas and get light relief without discomfort. If some jets bubble out of the floor of a pool, it feels especially restorative to massage the soles of your feet.

Bonus Question: What should you NOT have done in your 26point2?

Don't show up to a marathon with unorganized tech! For example, if you are planning on listening to music at some point in your run, make sure to have a playlist cued up and easily accessible. During the Slovenian Radenci Marathon, around the 18-mile mark (30 km), I found myself running through country fields, with the sun high overhead, no shade and no runners in sight to chat with. I was fading and needed a boost. Energetic music seemed to be just the answer. However, in my haste to arrive to the destination race, I hadn't properly organized my running playlist. I found myself slowing down to fiddle with my phone, first to locate music that was already downloaded, and then to sift through the available songs to find my favorite high-energy ones.

When a song was over, inevitably a slower song I was less enthusiastic about would follow and I'd have to take my phone out again to search for a better option. I lost precious minutes during the searches and ended up giving up the music altogether shortly after. The only bright side to this rookie mistake was that when attempting to access the music on my phone, I saw a text flash on the screen from fellow runner Sarah (featured in Chapter 15!) with her wishes that I finish well and enjoy a celebratory beer afterward. Since I hadn't planned on looking at my phone at all during the race, it was extra special to see her message at that moment. I felt her enthusiastic support beaming to me from another country while I was alone in the middle of nowhere, and it left a smile on my face and lightened my step.

And yes, I was able to find an excellent Slovenian beer as she had hoped, and it was even served with popcorn! I am not usually a beer drinker, but many marathoners agree that a cold beer definitely hits the spot shortly after crossing the finish line of a 26point2. Additionally, as if in a movie, the hot sunny day dramatically shifted and just as I raised my celebratory glass, the skies opened up to release a refreshing rain shower that lasted about five minutes. The perfect punctuation to a great race!

***

Mary Anne N., from USA, has run in USA, Australia, Austria, Bolivia, Canada, China (in the Great Wall Marathon!), Costa Rica, Croatia, the Czech Republic, Germany, Greece, Guatemala, Honduras, Hungary, Indonesia, Lithuania, Malta, Mexico, Panama, Portugal, Peru, Senegal, Slovakia, Slovenia, South Korea, Spain, Switzerland, and Thailand

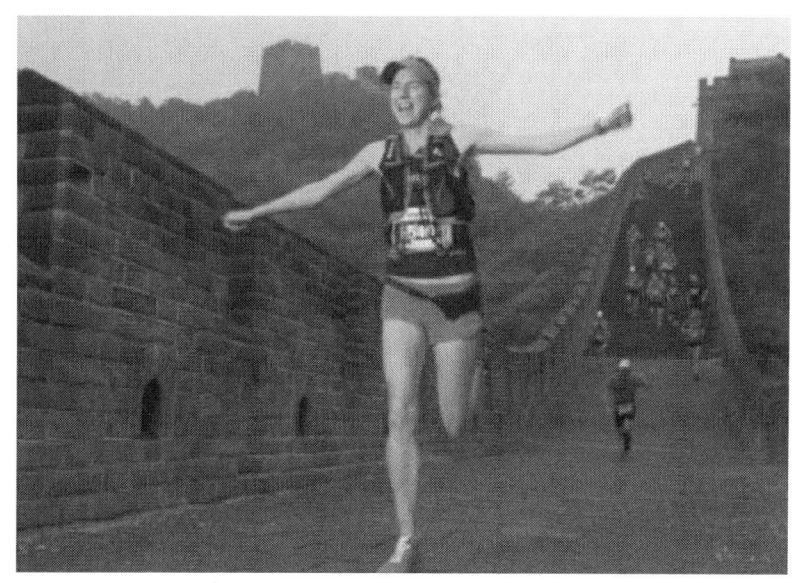

Mary Anne on the run of a lifetime: 26point2 on the Great Wall of China! (Photo from Marathon-Photo)

Mile 0.2: What NOT to Do While Racing in a Marathon: The Chicken Pudding 0.2 Interview

Juan S. from Taiwan

In order to round out the 26point2 interviews, I reached out to international runner Juan S. for a mini 0.2 interview, which we did over a light Sunday jog. While the overarching theme of this book involves ideas you can use to enhance and improve your marathon experience, Juan's story can be filed under the "What NOT to do" category. He was kind enough to share his story to alert other runners to a few things they can do to avoid similar missteps.

Juan has a fascinating multicultural background. He hails from Taiwan originally but has called Argentina, USA, Austria, and Chile home. He has run the streets of many international cities, and when he heard of a truly singular marathon race experience in Istanbul, Turkey, he decided it was a must-try event to add to his growing list of running adventures.

The reason this particular race caught Juan's attention is that runners embark on an intercontinental route. Istanbul straddles both Asia and Europe, and the marathon route takes runners over a massive bridge that connects one continent to the other to reach the finish line. This is the only marathon in the world that can claim a continental crossover by land.

Finishing a race route that spans two continents is quite a feather for any runner's hat, and Juan was up for the challenge.

He made two attempts to take on this iconic race, yet we will hope that the third time's the charm as his first two efforts lead to DNFs (Did Not Finish results). The two disappointments, caused by unforeseen circumstances, are things that all runners can learn from, especially when trying out a race in a far-flung destination.

Turkey: Take One

While reading this book, one might ask how Juan and others like him are able to country hop the world racing in diverse and unusual locations. There are many ways to do this. Study abroad students, digital nomads, foreign service employees, and traveling business professionals are among the many international racers I have come across that can lace up their shoes in various countries throughout the year. Another contingent includes people involved with the international school system.

International schools typically serve the children of embassy workers from around the world, United Nations employees, and people from other global organizations. Teachers at these schools are often expats themselves and enjoy frequent mini breaks in addition to long summer and winter holidays. They are therefore likely to be seasoned world travelers. The only caveat is that the travel must fall neatly within the designated school breaks, and there is little to no flexibility within the academic calendar.

Due to this tight scheduling, Juan, an international school science teacher, attempted to book his Istanbul 26point2 weekend around his school schedule. On the day of his flight, the commute time from the school to the airport train station was cut a bit too close. Upon missing the first train to the airport, he caught the next one and made his way to the check-in counter while dodging other travelers and their luggage. He felt much like a marathoner just over the starting line darting around the jumbled mass of people.

Alas, he arrived at his flight counter with only twenty minutes before his plane was due to take off, and the airline employee was unwilling to let him attempt boarding. This was even after he explained that he was, in fact, traveling for a marathon and could absolutely run to reach his plane before the gate closed. Due to time constraints and the financial considerations involved with catching the next flight out, he decided to defer his intercontinental marathon experience to the following year.

Turkey: Take Two

Fast forward to the next year and Juan had again trained for the same marathon in Turkey. This time he was at the airport before his flight to Istanbul with plenty of time to enjoy a relaxing coffee before take-off. He gave himself such a wide berth before the start of the race that he was able to take in the running Expo before the event and even donated a sapling to keep the parks of Istanbul green for generations of runners to come.

Juan had time to leisurely wander around the city before his race, exploring the vibrant culture of Turkey among the minarets and domes of the ancient streets. Many travelers feel the drive to follow their taste buds, and sampling local dishes becomes a priority when visiting a new city. Juan decided to try some traditional foods despite his plan to run the marathon the day after his city tour. One dish that stood out with him is known as Turkish chicken pudding.

Tavuk göğüsü is a traditional Turkish dessert that contains fine shreds of white chicken that are carefully strained into its flan-like texture. The dessert is sweet and has notes of cinnamon, yet it is also high-protein. It is a favorite at Turkish tea time.

Unfortunately, Juan did not have a positive experience with the dessert and is convinced that the chicken pudding he sampled the night before the marathon left him with a queasy and unsettled stomach the morning of the race. He felt weak and generally unwell but chose to run anyway. After all, he was so happy that he had made his flight to Istanbul that he had to give it a shot!

As Juan made his way through the stunning course that wound through the city, he started feeling awful and was worried he would be sick in the middle of the race. Therefore, when he passed by the door of his hotel right on the racecourse, he made the quick decision to pull out of the marathon. He spent the remainder of his visit to Istanbul sick in his hotel room.

I hope to catch Juan in Turkey for "take three" of his Istanbul racing attempts and finish this iconic race with him. I'm sure that when he finally does reach the finish line, after that incredible intercontinental crossing, his victory will be even sweeter than the fateful chicken pudding. He has learned from his past attempts and when he looks to do this marathon again, he will no doubt save the sampling of exotic dishes for a post-race celebration. No matter how enticing local cuisine may be, **it's better not to try new adventures in dining before a 26point2**.

***

Juan S., from Taiwan, has run in Austria, Chile, Turkey, and USA

26point2 Tips & Tweaks

The following are small ideas gleaned from runners around the world. Give them a try if you'd like, and please note that some are country-specific and relevant only in certain contexts:

1. (Used in China) Consuming gels and drinking isotonic beverages on the run can lead to sticky hands for the duration of a race. One runner smartly slips a few individually wrapped moist towelettes into her waist pack and avoids the mess by wiping down after each gel or sports drink. Just be sure not to litter the wrappers and used towelettes.

2. (Used in the UK) When participating in a destination marathon race, investigate in advance what the aid stations will provide. One runner inquires ahead, and if the offerings are unfamiliar to her, she'll order the product online first to test it out while training.

3. (Used in USA) Get friendly with your (not so nearby) neighbors and let them know in advance that you will drop some water bottles off on their property before long training runs and perhaps shed a layer of clothing and leave it there (to be picked up later) as well. That way, you can count on hydration even when far from home and be more comfortable if you happen to overdress. If you freeze the bottles before dropping them off, they should still be cold when you drink them.

4. (Used in Dubai, UAE) Map out your available hydration stations on long runs (clearly of high concern while marathon training in a country with extreme temperatures and sandstorms!) and note the accessible places for bathroom breaks.

5. (All over) If you are doing a destination marathon in a country where you are unfamiliar with the language, bring a

supply of sample-size creams you might need (for example, petroleum jelly or a topical muscle pain relief ointment) and carry these in a waist belt. You may not recognize or be able to read the labels if local brands are offered. One marathoner reported accidentally accepting the wrong cream while racing abroad. He used a stinging topical ointment on an open chafing wound instead of the soothing cream he believed it to be. The use of the wrong product made an already uncomfortable situation extremely painful.

6. (Used in Honduras) Scatter small coins when out on a training run and remember where you placed them. You can make a game of guessing if they will still be there or not the next time you run, and if they are gone you can make up a story in your head about what might have happened to them.

7. (Used in Spain, and all over) The workout app Aaptive has been helpful for many up-and-coming marathoners to progressively build up their running foundation with music and other motivational workouts that guide you towards the goal of a successful 26point2.

8. (Used in Austria) Borrow from the babes and take mini pure fruit bars in portions meant for toddlers along on your runs or races. These individually packaged snacks made of different fruit combinations are roughly the size of a postage stamp. A full-size bar is not always needed and these smaller alternatives provide a convenient bite of energy. It's never ideal to carry a sticky half-eaten bar in your running gear. The HiPP brand has a nice selection of flavors (www.hipp.com).

9. (Used in Los Angeles, USA) Get a professional stretch after your race day or integrate them into the training plan. Runners seek out places such as Stretch Lab (www.stretchlab.com) where professional stretchers called Flexologists specialize in reducing pain in sore and tight areas by literally stretching you out with their techniques.

10. (Used in Thailand) Foot massages, lasting from 30 to

90 minutes, can be a distance runner's best friend, especially when added to marathon preparation and recovery. Thai-style massages are particularly effective and provide a release in the tension of the fascia band, which can be key to preventing injury in this area. Some believe that certain pressure points on the foot will release tension in corresponding parts of the body as well.

     11. (Used in Ethiopia) Acupuncture can be highly effective in treating various running-related injuries. One runner reported getting treatment for IT band issues from an acupuncturist in Ethiopia, which helped to reduce tightness and inflammation. Many find this to be an effective therapy to relieve ongoing running injuries.

     12. (Seen in China) In China, it is not unusual for runners to light up a celebratory cigarette immediately after the race, so anyone wishing to steer clear of smoke after their run should plan on leaving the finish line area.

     13. (Used in Malaysia and Thailand) In some countries, race start times might take place well before sunrise to avoid steamy running conditions. Prepare to be an early bird and expect extremely early start times. When factoring in travel time, breakfast and warming up, a 3:30 a.m. wakeup call, or even earlier, might be necessary on race day. The Bangkok Marathon in Thailand is an extreme example of the pre-dawn approach and starts at midnight. Runners should adjust their race preparations accordingly.

     14. (Used in USA) Share the glory of winning a medal with someone suffering from a severe health issue. There is a program called Medals4Mettle in which marathoners donate their race medals to children and adults that struggle with cancer, other illnesses, or trauma. The idea behind this gesture is to award the strength and courage of the person suffering a health challenge. One runner I know has even met the young patient that this program sends her medals to in person and thinks of

the joy she will give her friend with each new medal won. This generous act provides deep motivation for the runner and compassion and encouragement for the recipient of the medal. See www.medals4mettle.org for more information.

    15. (Used in South Africa) In big races in South Africa, runners report that it is not uncommon to proudly pin a badge on your race day gear that states your age. A race spectator noted that, "It was incredible to support runners in their 70s, 80s, and 90s. They were whizzing by with the biggest smiles on their faces."

    16. (Used in USA) Marathons have finish times that shut the race down and force runners that do not end in time to resign to a dreaded DNF (Did Not Finish) result. To avoid this, one back-of-the-pack runner calculates the time she needs for each segment of the race in order get to the finish line before it closes. She makes an Excel chart of the necessary splits and then cleverly saves this chart as the screen saver of her cell phone. This way, she has her cheat sheet readily available and doesn't need to open her phone and dig around for it during the race. She also sets alarms on her phone to go off at her target 10-km, 20-km, and 30-km times, so she can check if she's on track.

    17. (Used in Russia) Take special note of the extraordinary advantages found only on race day. One runner in Moscow could not put her finger on what was so different about her home city during her 26point2. She finally realized she had never in her life seen the wide-open avenues and glorious sights in her hometown *without any traffic*. She made a point to soak up this luxury as the city is almost always congested with cars. In awe, she saw her home with new eyes and finished the race with a deep appreciation of places she had seen, but not really noticed before.

    18. (Used in Aruba) Those that suffer from plantar fasciitis know about a prevention and treatment technique that uses a cylinder to roll out this thick, web-like ligament.

Rolling provides immediate relief and loosens up the area significantly, but not all foot rolling devices are created equally. Enter the TenderFoot Therapeutic roller.

An athletic family that I know graciously shared the TenderFoot with me. They learned about it in Aruba, where they met its creator. I was suffering from a massive injury to the fascia, and by introducing me to the TenderFoot, this family greatly facilitated my recovery process. Years later, I am still grateful for this gesture and blissfully roll out as often as possible.

Weighing in at 3.5 pounds (1.59 kilos), this squat roller made of blue aluminum features a knurled surface. This texture, along with the substantial weight of the roller, allows for excellent controlled rolling and noticeable relief to precise points of tension. It is the Rolls Royce of foot rollers and comes with a price tag to match, but it gets impressive results.

There is a limited quantity of TenderFoot rollers produced because, as mentioned, the price point is steep for this kind of product. That said, for those runners that struggle with ongoing plantar fasciitis issues, it is an excellent investment (more information can be obtained by writing to tfinfo@tenderfootinc.com).

19. (Used in Austria) Take Red Bull off the dance floor and put it on the racecourse. The Red Bull energy beverage has its roots in Thailand and made its way to Europe where it's now sold by an Austrian company. In some parts of the world you might only see Red Bull in a cocktail glass with vodka added to it, but in Austria, the slim blue and silver can is spotted all around, including in the hands of distance runners. As one marathoner stated, "I love Red Bull because it is not sweet, it raises my energy level, and has little bubbles which make it nice to drink during the race."

20. (Used in Austria) Repurpose your accessories to suit your running needs. One marathoner, frustrated with inevit-

ably losing an expensive pair of thin running gloves every winter, impulsively threw a pair of cotton socks on her hands one brisk morning and discovered her new favorite "running mittens." Using inexpensive socks as mittens is one effective way to cope with colder weather since they are comfortable and if you lose them over the course of the run, it is not a major loss.

21. (Used in Malaysia) If you are peppering road races throughout your marathon training cycle, in some places it's necessary to closely study the event calendar and register for the race as quickly as possible. In the US, for example, it's very common to impulsively join a road race the morning of the event and sign up on-site (albeit for a slightly higher fee, but the option often exists). This is not necessarily the case in other countries, including Malaysia, where races sell out very quickly and it's therefore necessary to register as early as possible.

21. (Used in Cambodia) People vary on how they feel about this practice, but some runners racing in developing countries like to bring along small trinkets or stickers to hand out to young kids in the crowd cheering them on. This gesture is to thank them for their support and simply create a small connection.

23. (Used in USA) Make training runs a game by involving kids. It's often a challenge for parents to juggle childcare responsibilities within a marathon training cycle. Bringing kids along helps; small children can ride in streamlined jogging strollers that have good suspension systems, and older kids can use their bikes to keep up. Sometimes, however, it takes a little creative incentive so that restless little ones enjoy the ride. One marathoner shared, "I created a game for my daughter. She would bike while I ran. If she saw a turtle, she would get $1.00 and a bunny $0.50, and so on. She is now 13 and still tries to play and get money from me!"

24. (Used in France) Even if you run in an urban area,

embrace the trail running backpack. You can remove the hydration bladders from these multipurpose accessories to carry anything you might need on a long run such as energy bars, sports drinks, headphones, phone, keys, wallet, and extra layers of non-bulky clothes. It can also serve as a portable cosmetics case/toiletry bag if you convert your commute into a training session and run to work. A good quality trail backpack will fit snuggly to your body, so it won't bounce when running.

25. (Used in Sweden) A Swedish marathoner shared that blueberry soup is excellent for race refueling. Traditionally served at Vasaloppet, the world's most historic cross-country ski race, blueberry soup or *Blåbärssoppa* is a versatile refueling option. It can be served hot in cold weather (many racers carry it around in thermoses) or cold in warm weather. The berries are cooked with sugar and potato starch for a boost of fast-acting energy and it "Amazingly hits the spot after a hard run," reports the runner.

26. (Used in Japan) A runner from Tokyo explained why a treat called Mochi that is traditional for the Japanese New Year is her go-to for running fuel. "Mochi is pounded steamed rice, so the final product is highly condensed pure carb. I'll eat about three or four before going out." It's said that this was also what samurai warriors ate before battle for stamina!

.2 (Used all over) JUST HAVE FUN! Don't forget to take it all in! Running forces you to be in the moment. Enjoy the context of your run; note the sky, the time of day, the season, and the sites around you. Many of the runners featured in this book are lucky enough to make incredible world experiences a part of their running. Whether you happen to be racing through lava fields in Iceland, on the Great Wall of China, or on a bridge in Istanbul crossing from one continent to the next (or simply on your local street that has an iconic status in your personal life!), take a meaningful moment to appreciate the surroundings. No matter where you are or how hard the run is, remind yourself to be grateful to be able to do it.

Looking Ahead

The book in your hands is a stepping stone to something bigger. The first edition of *Around the Globe in 26point2 Miles* will serve to get the word out about the heart of this project which is sharing running ideas from around the world. There is perhaps too much of a focus on certain regions, and not enough attention is given to other, less accessible areas. This is not due to lack of interest; it's just a reflection of the first ring of people I've been able to connect with through my running contacts, and their kind and willing friends around the world.

Therefore, the idea is that *Around the Globe in 26point2 Miles* will expand and evolve to include new regions of the world and other cultures! The first 26point2 interviews are simply a starting point to continue building on. My aim is to connect with new runners and reach 42.195 interviews the next time around, including both new and other well-known voices in the world of marathoners. The final result will ideally be a pictorial celebration of these shared findings in the form of a coffee table-style book that one can hold, flip through, and turn to time and time again for inspiration.

All new running-related ideas and experiences are welcome for the upcoming project *Around the Globe in 42point195 Kilometers*. There are also specific voices I am hoping will respond and share, such as:

--Scott Jurek, on how a vegan diet can lead to outstanding marathon training.

--Haile Gebrselassie, on how to train like a local at the Yaya Village in Ethiopia. How do popcorn and coffee come into play?

--Queen Oprah Winfrey, walking us through her marathon debut at the Marine Corps Marathon in USA.

--"Mr. Great Wall" Henrik Brandt, author of *If You Can Dream It You Can Do It*, on how he went from a couch potato to the only person in the world who has run all 20 years of the Great Wall Marathons (the most recent ones after having a pacemaker implanted).

--Yuki Kawauchi on embracing the fun element of marathons (including the use of costumes) while still getting phenomenal times.

--Pippa Middleton, future marathon mama, on her top experiences while racing around the world.

--Desi Linden on coffee, whiskey and 26.2 brew in the champion running equation.

--Eliud Kipchoge on his historic success while using the Maurten beverage, the perks of drinking two liters of tea a day, and what's going through his mind before he come to Vienna this year in a historic attempt to break the two-hour marathon barrier.

--Dave Heely on running blind with a guide runner and the incredible accomplishment of completing seven marathons in seven days spanning seven continents.

--Team Goop on incorporating clean fueling into marathon training.

--Manuel Luna on the details behind the extraordinary running endurance of the Tarahumara in Copper Canyon.

--Jamdammers Jamaican marathoners about the Reggae Marathon experience and how sweet potatoes form part of running nutrition.

International marathoners around the world: what inspires your running and what culturally-based elements go into your 26point2 experience? Please reach out and share at: aroundtheglobein26point2miles@gmail.com. Thank you!

Acknowledgments

Here's the Oscars Speech:

Many people went into the making of this book! With sincere gratitude, I'd like to thank the 26 runners that graciously participated in my interviews. Your words are the cornerstone of this project; thank you for bringing me along on your unique marathon experiences. From Queenie, Janelle, Baláz, Diane, Mihnea, Julio A., Juan, Sandeep, Johanna, Lia, Jesper, Julio M.C., Alastair, Christine, Togz, Sarah, Ben, Kristin, Ina, Iván, Jean-Marie, Željko, Peter, Diana, Emmanuelle, and Becky, I've learned that runners are a unique breed and the best bunch of people you could hope to learn from. Thanks also go to the many others that have contributed insight, inspiration, connections and tips for this book (including Natalia, Sally, Lisa, Tini & Renée, Sherri, Connie, Stacie, Mika, Tova, Sasha, Annie, Katie, Jenn, Dr. Liz, and Emy).

To all my running friends from around the world, and to all that put me in touch with international runners, thank you. I would like to namely thank my running families: *Los Jartibles*, in Sevilla, and the Sunday B'run'chers (Group TGV) in Vienna.

The 2013 marathon in Sevilla provided most of the basis for Chapter 26. I want to thank everyone who was along for the ride during that singular experience, especially: "Coach Espi" Jose Manuel; Pepe "Footing" Fotos and family; "Presi Coco" Jose Antonio and family; and Paco Esteban, Dani Q., Francisco (the photographer), and IMD Sevilla.

I'm grateful to friends that have given their local and long-distance support to this project, including Christie, who helped with the initial brainstorming years ago over tapas, and *mis Americanitas*.

Thank you to my dad and siblings and Uncle Greg for being supportive and true examples of resilience in the marathon of life! An extra special thank you to my dad, just because he is the best. He climbed the Acropolis in extreme heat, and his support means everything.

There are not enough words left in the world to thank a pure ray of sunshine that waits for me at finish lines in different countries and patiently (some of the time!) logs miles with me in the jogging stroller. Lola Q., thank you for putting up with a mom that takes you running through the vineyards, and eventually wants to take you to the Himalayas, among other future adventures! And most of all, to Jman, who always believes. You're supportive of every adventure and sometimes even thank me for going on my own (Gracias por irte :) jaja). I owe you all my gratitude — you already have all of my heart. (Ok... Pouffa...thank you too).

About the Author

    I'm a runner and world wanderer who was named poster woman of the marathon in Sevilla, Spain, due to my cultural duality as a Minnesotan who has spent half her life abroad. The idea behind Sevilla's marathon campaign that year was to highlight the international spirit that the 26point2 promotes. I embrace the connection that running grants people from different backgrounds. To me, one of the best feelings in the world is stepping on the soil of at least one new country per year (hopefully more!) and if, at all possible, getting a run in among the locals. In doing so, I've met some incredible people, discovered unique running rituals and training aspects, and I've also caught some spectacular sunrises. All of this forms the foundation of *Around the Globe in 26point2 Miles*.

Thank you for reading and happy running!
M.A. Nixon
2019

Printed in Poland
by Amazon Fulfillment
Poland Sp. z o.o., Wrocław